THE NEW HEALTH POLICY

STATE OF HEALTH SERIES

Edited by Chris Ham, Professor of Health Policy and Management at the University of Birmingham and Director of the Strategy Unit at the Department of Health.

Current and forthcoming titles

THE NEW HEALTH POLICY

Robin Gauld

Open University Press

Open University Press
McGraw-Hill Education
McGraw-Hill House
Shoppenhangers Road
Maidenhead
Berkshire
England
SL6 2QL

email: enquiries@openup.co.uk
world wide web: www.openup.co.uk

and Two Penn Plaza, New York, NY 10121-2289, USA

First published 2009

A catalogue record of this book is available from the British Library

ISBN-13: 978-0-33-522903-1 (pb) 978-0-33-522902-4 (hb)
ISBN-10: 033522903 4 (pb) 033522902 6 (hb)

Library of Congress Cataloging-in-Publication Data
CIP data applied for

Typeset by RefineCatch Limited, Bungay, Suffolk
Printed in the UK by Bell and Bain Ltd, Glasgow.

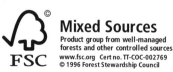

Mixed Sources
Product group from well-managed
forests and other controlled sources
www.fsc.org   Cert no. TT-COC-002769
© 1996 Forest Stewardship Council

FSC

The McGraw·Hill Companies

CONTENTS

ACKNOWLEDGEMENTS

Book writing does not happen without the assistance of various people. I am therefore enormously grateful to Chris Ham for supporting this book project and providing comments on earlier drafts. I'm grateful also to Open University Press for their support and encouragement from when the book proposal was first put to them, through to the finished manuscript and, of course, the publication process. Initial drafts of the book were written in Dunedin, New Zealand, at the University of Otago; the final draft of the book was completed while I was on leave from Otago, based at Boston University's Health Policy Institute as a Commonwealth Fund Harkness Fellow. I am indebted to these organizations for their backing. The biggest debt, however, is to my family, who weathered the storm of writing. Thank you, Ina, Ted and Honor. This book is dedicated to you.

Robin Gauld
Lexington, Massachusetts
January, 2009

SERIES EDITOR'S INTRODUCTION

Health services in many developed countries have come under critical scrutiny in recent years. In part this is because of increasing expenditure, much of it funded from public sources, and the pressure this has put on governments seeking to control public spending. Also important has been the perception that resources allocated to health services are not always deployed in an optimal fashion. Thus at a time when the scope for increasing expenditure is extremely limited, there is a need to search for ways of using existing budgets more efficiently. A further concern has been the desire to ensure access to health care of various groups on an equitable basis. In some countries this has been linked to a wish to enhance patient choice and to make service providers more responsive to patients as consumers.

Underlying these specific concerns are a number of more fundamental developments which have a significant bearing on the performance of health services. Three are worth highlighting. First, there are demographic changes, including the ageing population and the decline in the proportion of the population of working age. These changes will both increase the demand for health care and at the same time limit the ability of health services to respond to this demand.

Second, advances in medical science will also give rise to new demands within the health services. These advances cover a range of possibilities, including innovations in surgery, drug therapy, screening and diagnosis. The pace of innovation quickened as the end of the twentieth century approached, with significant implications for the funding and provision of services.

Third, public expectations of health services are rising as those who use services demand higher standards of care. In part, this is stimulated by developments within the health service, including the availability of new technology. More fundamentally, it stems from the emergence of a more educated and informed population, in which people are accustomed to being treated as consumers rather than patients.

Against this background, policy makers in a number of countries are reviewing the future of health services. Those countries which have traditionally relied on a market in health care are making greater use of regulation and planning. Equally, those countries which have traditionally relied on regulation and planning are moving towards a more competitive approach. In no country is there complete satisfaction with existing methods of financing and delivery, and everywhere there is a search for new policy instruments.

The aim of this series is to contribute to debate about the future of health services through an analysis of major issues in health policy. These issues have been chosen because they are both of current interest and of enduring importance. The series is intended to be accessible to students and informed lay readers as well as to specialists working in this field. The aim is to go beyond a textbook approach to health policy analysis and to encourage authors to move debate about their issues forward. In this sense, each book presents a summary of current research and thinking, and an exploration of future policy directions.

Professor Chris Ham
Professor of Health Policy and Management at the University of Birmingham

ABBREVIATIONS

AHRQ	Agency for Healthcare Research and Quality
CHC	Community Health Council
CQI	continuous quality improvement
DHB	District Health Board
EHR	electronic health record
GMC	General Medical Council
HAZ	Health Action Zones
ICT	Information and Communications Technology
ISTC	independent sector treatment centre
LINKs	Local Involvement Networks
MSA	medical savings account
MDGs	Millennium Development Goals
NICE	National Institute for Health and Clinical Excellence
NPSA	National Patient Safety Agency
OECD	Organization for Economic Cooperation and Development
PCT	Primary Care Trust
PFI	Private Finance Initiative
PHO	Primary Health Organization
PSO	Patient Safety Organization
WHO	World Health Organization

1

INTRODUCTION

From around the early 1980s, various developed world governments commenced a process of reforming their health care policies and systems. This 'reform era' has been widely studied and written about, with particular regard to the fact that there was something of a common agenda. A central tenet of this agenda was the application of neoliberal, or market-oriented, philosophies to drive policy development and service organization (Walsh 1995; Altenstetter and Bjorkman 1997; Callahan and Wasunna 2006). Stemming from this, governments opted for competitive models of organization, for private-sector influenced managerial and funding arrangements, and for clear limits on the role of the state in health care funding and delivery.

The 'reform era' agenda appeared to be in descent by around the mid–late 1990s or so as a range of new ideas about health policy, health system structure and service delivery have made their way onto the global policy agenda and that of national governments. These ideas were in recognition of various difficulties with the reform era, and of new thinking about and research into how best to organize health systems and improve their performance in the face of growing demand and costs, advancing technology, ageing populations and concerns about quality. The ideas were also driven by the ascendence of social democratic and related political philosophies (Giddens 1998).

However, to suggest that there is a new social democratic agenda may be to oversimplify the national and global patterns of health policy and service delivery structures in place today. Indeed, underpinning policies and service organization in many countries can be found the hallmarks of neoliberalism. These have often been reasserted behind policies that appear to be designed to improve collaboration and participation in health care decision making and delivery, and to establish the presence of the state with an apparently genuine concern about and responsibility for health care and public health improvement. The result has been a complex diversity of health reforms and structures for governance and service delivery that includes the use of market mechanisms and the private sector, of government agencies and bureaucracies, and of network organizational arrangements. It has also meant a changing role for the main actors in the health sector including the state, the private sector, the professions and the public.

This book is about health policy developments in this era of complexity. It discusses a series of policy issues that are central to the agendas of developed world governments today, and looks at how, in practical terms, different countries have responded. It looks at the mix of policies and at the differing organizational structures that have emerged. In this regard, the book analyses the hub of what is referred to as the 'new health policy'.

The topics covered in the book are drawn from a potentially vast list, such is the nature and complexity of health care delivery and policy. Each of the core chapters considers what is a key concern of national governments and international agencies such as the World Health Organization (WHO) and the Organization for Economic Cooperation and Development (OECD). These core chapters cover the nucleus of the new health policy agenda. Absent are chapters on issues such as primary care, rationing and the role of the hospital that are also high on the international policy agenda. These topics are covered in passing but the decision not to specifically focus on them is intentional as they have been substantially covered elsewhere (for example, McKee and Healy 2002; Ham and Robert 2003; Jost 2004; Saltman et al. 2006; World Health Organization 2008). Each of the core chapters also discusses practical approaches to the policy issues in different countries. The primary focus is on Britain, with New Zealand and the US also emphasized for comparison. To further illustrate certain issues, other country examples are periodically discussed.

This introductory chapter has two aims. First, it backgrounds the context within which the new health policy has emerged. The following section therefore outlines the above-mentioned theories that have underpinned policy developments, namely neoliberalism and social democracy. It provides a general overview of the emerging patterns of policy and the organizational forms found in health systems today. It then discusses key practical issues driving the new health policy agenda, including increasing service demand and expenditure, new diseases and health risks, demographic change, and quality concerns. The final section addresses the second aim of the chapter, which is to overview the remainder of the book.

THE CONTEXT FOR THE NEW HEALTH POLICY

Political philosophies driving health policy

The 'health reform era' spanning a decade from around the mid-1980s to the mid-1990s saw health systems throughout the world subject to radical neoliberal-inspired reform efforts. Governments have since, however, continued to focus on health system reforms influenced by a mix of neoliberal and social democratic concepts in what is termed here the 'post-reform era'. The following sections overview the influence of neoliberalism in the reform era and then social democracy in the post-reform era.

The 'reform era': neoliberalism

Neoliberal theory encapsulated a series of ideas which, combined, amounted to an attack on pre-existing government and public services. These arrangements tended to include central planning and administration of health systems, and leadership at the service delivery level by medical and other health professionals.

The health reform era commenced around the mid-1980s prompted by increasing concern at growing health care costs, as well as neoliberal philosophy. As Ham notes, there were essentially three components of the neoliberal approach (Ham 1997: 8–9). First was that systems required the forces of private markets to improve their efficiency and increase the range of services available. Driving this was a belief that central planners were incapable of producing ideas for health system improvement. Also, however, several countries in the mid-1980s elected right-wing governments with a preference for markets, public sector downsizing and privatization. The preference for markets saw the creation of purchasers and providers, and the introduction of contracting between these two parties, within previously integrated hierarchical health systems. Of course, in tandem with the purchaser-provider split, many countries reformed the organization of health care delivery. This included creating new corporate structures to manage hospitals and requirements that publicly-owned and/or funded agencies compete with one another.

Second, and in keeping with 'managerialism', was a desire to implement robust health services management systems. This was propelled by perceptions that health professionals lacked appropriate expertise in management, such as experience in running private business, and were incapable of making objective managerial decisions due to their allegiances with professional colleagues. Improved management also required an orientation toward 'customers', dedication to improved service performance through developing workforce objectives and incentives and devolving responsibility for these to appropriate units, and a focus on contracting out of services to induce competition and reduce costs. Very importantly, it required a concerted effort to improve performances in areas such as hospital average length of stay, waiting times for elective treatments, and health outcomes. To empower and provide incentives for improved hospital and other local service management, such responsibilities were decentralized. This meant that budgetary, human resource and service organization decisions were a managerial responsibility and largely separate from central government intervention.

Third was the reform of budgetary systems and creation of financial incentives to improve performance. A core idea, applied across government systems, was that funding ought to be oriented toward 'outputs and outcomes' instead of simply based on prior expenditure and utilization patterns. Thus, policy makers required that providers develop information systems as well as methods for micro-managing workforce activities. This was so that funders (or purchasers) would be able to see exactly what they were paying for. They would also be able to see how these activities were contributing to desired policy outcomes (long term health policy objectives).

Various other budgeting and funding initiatives were developed in the reform era. These included prospective global budgets, an annual sum of money paid over to a provider who would then carry responsibility for cost over-runs. Global budgets were also applied to purchasing (commissioning) agencies. These proved effective in areas such as drug buying. For example, New Zealand's Pharmaceutical Management Agency, formed in the early-1990s, used its purchasing power to drive down prices of publicly-purchased prescription drugs. This, combined with other strategies, allowed it to keep within budget. To provide incentives to improve service efficiency and quality, diagnostic related group funding methods emerged. These pay a fixed sum for pre-determined procedures (for example, birth by caesarian section), as opposed to paying for each individual provider and process involved, and can feature incentives for performance improvements. Finally, patient charges for public services were introduced as a revenue generator and to stem patient demand in the assumption that if people have to pay for health care they will think carefully about whether they really need to seek treatment.

The 'post-reform' era: social democracy

The post-reform era equates broadly with a general swing in politics away from neoliberalism and toward social democracy. In practice, in the health policies of most developed nations there is now a mix of neoliberal and social democratic influence. This is partly a function of the emergence of governments that are neither 'left' nor 'right' of the political spectrum but aim to occupy the centre ground, appealing to the middle classes as well as lower socio-economic groups, business and the wealthy. This centrist orientation has allowed for continuation of neoliberal ideas and institutions, while in pursuit of social democratic objectives. It is also a function of 'path dependency' (Wilsford 1994). This is where governments inherit institutional arrangements that are often strongly embedded and difficult to break free from and so policy tends to consist of adjustments to existing foundations.

Social democratic philosophy, which was behind the public policies of many western nations in the post-war, pre-neoliberal era, drove many of the ideas of Bill Clinton's Democratic Presidency in the United States (1993–2001), as well as those of Tony Blair's New Labour government (1997–2007). Social democracy has long provided the foundation for governments in Western Europe and Scandinavia (Paterson and Thomas 1986; Milner 1990). While neoliberalism might be considered a 'hard' worldview, social democracy could be seen by its very nature as softer in that it is focused on both 'society' and 'democracy'. Social democracy is guided by a range of ideas (see generally Giddens 1998).

First, that there is a very definite role for the state in developing a robust and caring society. A particular focus is on humanitarian principles of ensuring that all people have access to basic goods and services. Thus, social democrats may argue for state intervention in the 'supply-side' of the economy if this is not providing for the needs of all – something that neoliberals refrain from. A social democratic government will probably make sure that education is freely and universally available, along with health care, housing and a reasonable minimum income level. There may be additional benefits and services for the less well off and for certain groups such as the elderly and disadvantaged minorities who have demonstrated needs. The social democratic tradition was heavily influenced by the Great Depression of the 1930s, when many people suffered severe hardship. The resulting suffering was subsequently viewed as avoidable with state assistance. Social democracy is, therefore, equated with the development of the welfare state and also with interventionist, Keynesian economics (Leijonhufvud 1968).

Second, despite its 'social' foundations, the capitalist economy is central to social democratic principles. It is viewed as the most appropriate and effective form of organization. The role of government is to promote a humane variant of capitalism. A key aim, therefore, is to develop an economy with people at the centre. Regulations will be applied to uphold certain work conditions and payrates, there will be support for lower socio-economic groups and the unemployed, and government will invest in infrastructure and selected industries seen to be beneficial to the welfare of the economy and society.

Third, a liberal tradition within social democratic theory limits the extent to which a social democratic state will intervene in society and the economy. Classical liberalism, which neoliberalism drew upon, had at its core the idea that individuals and the economy should be as free as possible from state intervention. People and businesses should be able to pursue their own interests within the laws set down by the state, and have the freedom to openly express ideas and critique public policy. In the spirit of this, social democracy seeks to enhance freedoms and the free society.

Fourth, by definition, democratic government is at the centre of social democracy. This means that governments and representatives, at both the national and local levels of government, are elected through regular, free and transparent polls in which all eligible citizens have the right to participate and hold political leaders to account. It means that government ought to represent the will of the people and reflect this in policy-making, but also that maximum opportunity be provided for public consultation and deliberation through the policy process. Thus, in contrast with neoliberalism, where those in power may often view the public as misinformed and consultation will therefore be deemed irrelevant, there is a strong element of political pluralism within social democratic theory in that each member of society should have the capacity to contribute to the policy process.

Organizational forms: hierarchies, markets, networks and partnerships

There has been something of a transition through the post-war period in the organizational forms used for health care planning and delivery. The transition has, in many ways, reflected the dominant theories driving governments at different points in time, but also changing patterns and new developments in service delivery.

In the immediate post-war period, the hierarchical bureaucracy was the typical form for public service delivery. Bureaucracy has its roots in the process of industrialization and has been widely studied. Classic descriptions of bureaucracy can be found in the works of Max Weber who set out the characteristics of an organizational form centred around factories and offices. For Weber, a bureaucracy consisted of a hierarchical structure with a chain of workers divided into levels within the organization, each subservient and accountable to the one above it. Within each level, individual workers had specific tasks bounded by rules and limits on scope of practice and were arranged into departments or sections. The rules and control mechanisms were the hallmark of bureaucracy, with the written record the institutional memory. If a particular 'case' fell outside the boundaries of activity assigned to a worker, level or department, then it had to be referred to the appropriate area within the organization (Gerth and Mills 1948: 196–244).

While an effective form for its adherence to fairness, structure and division of labour into specialty group, bureaucracy has often been seen as inefficient as it takes time to process issues through different levels and workers within an entity (Wilson 1989). Moreover, in addition to the neoliberal critiques of government outlined above, bureaucracy has been challenged for its capacity for 'dehumanizing' both workers, who often lack power to undertake basic tasks outside their jurisdiction, and clients who are reduced to 'cases' that are moved about through an organization (Hummel 1987).

The large public hospital organization, of course, has often been considered a classic bureaucracy with separate departments organized around the many different medical specialties and services and a strict division of labour and structure for control within. Administrative leadership has traditionally been provided not by administrators but by health professionals, principally doctors and nurses. A

key aim of public hospital organizations within a public health system, such as in Britain, Hong Kong or New Zealand, is delivering
the range of essential through to advanced specialist services and
making these universally accessible.

The advent of neoliberalism has meant that market organizational
forms have become much more common for public health care
delivery (Flynn 1992; Hunter 1994). For public hospitals, this has
meant the removal of health professionals from leadership roles.
Replacing them have been generic managers, often especially
appointed because of experience in running private businesses.
Governments have also intentionally established mechanisms to
facilitate private services provision for public patients. Generally,
governments have used formal contracts for this by placing for open
tender specific public services to be delivered. Usually, these have
been non-urgent and routine services such as cataract surgery or hip
and knee joint replacements. This has been unpopular with public
providers with suggestions that such a move erodes public sector
capacity and potential to perform well, while providing incentives for
private providers to 'cream skim' the healthiest patients leaving the
public sector with the less well off and more difficult cases. Nonetheless, governments have often explicity cited a preference for private
provision under the assumption that this boosts competition, quality
and efficiency. Of course, because of cost there may be less incentive
for market-based organizations to provide high-tech advanced services that only a few patients will benefit from and have the ability to
pay for. A government will also have to pay close attention to regulating the standards of care provided. This is often where professional
bodies, such as the medical association and other workforce groups,
have an important role to play.

Gradual changes to the way in which health and other public
services are delivered have produced 'network' and 'partnership'
arrangements that are neither bureaucracy nor market (Thompson
et al. 1991). Networks may occur where a group of services providers, such as primary care physicians that work independently
from one another, are linked together. They may do so for information sharing, to ensure that a common population of patients are
appropriately catered to, or to share and distribute among one
another bulk funding from the government or another source. Thus,
a network is not necessarily about a preference for state or private
sector service delivery and neither is it defined by the walls of, say, a
hospital. A network may bring together providers with common
interests around serving patients with particular conditions and

therefore may include public, non-profit and private providers. Such a network may also involve patient or community representatives who are able to contribute to policy and service design and provide feedback. A network may be explicitly based on the idea of partnership where the providers jointly receive funding to deliver specified services. Crucial to such a partnership will be relationship building, collaboration and trust as well as a common interest in working together on an identified issue. A partnership may also be a simple case of a public organization, such as a hospital entering into a joint venture with a private or non-government provider or even a community to tackle a certain problem or develop a new programme to improve health.

Today, it is likely that all of the above organizational forms may be found. Large 'bureaucratic' public hospitals may subcontract some services such as non-urgent surgery to private providers. Public hospitals may find themselves in competition with private and non-government providers for contracts to provide publicly-funded services. There may be cases where public hospitals treat or provide specific services to private fee-paying patients, or provide different levels of care (such as single-occupancy rooms with higher quality cuisine) to patients prepared to pay a little extra. There may also be well-developed government-funded networks of public and private primary care practitioners that work in close partnership with their communities and public hospitals to improve the health care for their respective populations. Of course, in keeping with neoliberal notions, there may also be strong government incentives, including targets, for improving population health. This may even extend to empowering patient groups and the public per se – through a partnership arrangement where both state providers and the public are responsible for certain activities – so that they can produce health improving strategies and ultimately health. To the fore in such conditions may be health professionals and health promoters, given responsibility and held accountable for driving health improvement.

In parallel, a health policy agenda that favours devolution, accountability and democratic engagement with the community will most probably find such concepts represented in structures that hand responsibility for decision-making about local services delivery to localized governance structures. Such entities may have some freedom to implement policy, within government guidelines, as they see fit, but be subject to stringent accountability to and oversight by central government or a representative funding and monitoring institution. They may be required to consult widely and involve the community in processes of policy-making and service development. In this respect, service governance structures may extend to including community representatives. The 'community' may also include service providers and health professionals and so governance will closely involve such groups. In this way, a reemergence of health professional influence in management and decision-making may be facilitated, but with an emphasis on strong accountability.

Practical issues driving health policy

In addition to the political philosophies that have played a part in influencing health policy, a range of practical pressures and challenges are presently driving the agendas of the world's governments. Almost no developed world country is immune from these pressures, which are increasing over time, and each is developing means to deal with them. That said, solutions are not necessarily easily identifiable nor likely to fully alleviate the pressures. This section outlines the key practical issues facing developed world health systems today.

Demographic change and population ageing

Across the developed world there is mounting concern about declining rates of fertility, combined with increasing life expectancy. Figure 1.1 shows how fertility rates have dropped over time as measured by the number of children per woman. The data show that women in OECD countries are having fewer babies than they did in 1960. In most countries in the table the number of children per woman has dropped to well below the 2.1 requirement for population replacement. Partly, this is a function of a preference for smaller families, as well as the financial costs of having children and societal pressures on women to participate in the workforce and focus on career development. In practice, declining fertility means that the total population of affected countries is at risk of shrinking. With fewer children moving into adulthood, the longer-term implication is that the workforce will gradually diminish. This, in turn, means a declining tax base to pay for public services such as health care.

Declining fertility is occurring in tandem with increasing life expectancy across the developed world. People are living not only longer lives, but living for longer in retirement. OECD data show that the percentage of the population in member countries over 65 years (so called 'dependents') has grown from 8.9 in 1962 to 14.7

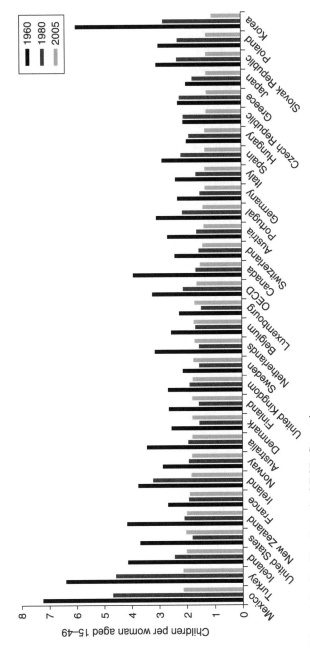

Figure 1.1 Fertility Rates in OECD Countries

Source: OECD (2007).

in 2005. Countries such as Japan, Italy and Germany have around 20 per cent in the over 65 group. Others with 'younger' populations including Turkey, Mexico and South Korea had less than 10 per cent over 65 in 2005, although the transition toward an older population is also well under way (OECD 2007). The trend of older populations is creating concern among policy makers in that they will require ever more money to fund an ever-expanding group of people with specific and often very costly health care needs. Declining fertility also means that there will be fewer family and other members of society to provide support for older people.

Increasing service demand and limited funding

Data show that, without exception, health care demand and expenditure in OECD member countries is increasing (see Figure 1.2). The 4 per cent OECD average increase in health expenditure shown in Figure 1.2 is well above the average 2.5 per cent average growth rate of OECD economies. In practice, this means that an increasing proportion of the economy, and in turn of the government budget, is being consumed by health care (OECD 2007). This trend is of concern to all affected countries and a common theme in reports by governments and international organizations. The key point made is that the rate of increase is 'unsustainable'.

The general consensus for dealing with this situation is that the options are to increase taxes and service funding, boost private funding of health services (insurance and point of service payments), improve the efficiency of health services and systems, or explicitly ration service access. Indeed, from around the early 1990s, 'rationing' and 'prioritization' have risen to the top of many government health policy agendas. Improving service efficiency has also been central to the rhetoric and actions of policy makers and managers. Yet reducing expenditure growth and service access are far from straightforward exercises which tend to be resisted by both the public and health professionals. In democratic societies, rationing and expenditure decisions can also be highly political.

Equally perplexing is determining what it is that is driving growth. Partly, it is the increasing scope of health systems and services as governments pursue new policies and health objectives. Expansion is also driven by technological advancements: the capacity to treat the previously untreatable, and the emergence of new drugs and therapies. Another driver is the expanding range of interventions available to patients seeking to enhance lifestyle, physical performance and

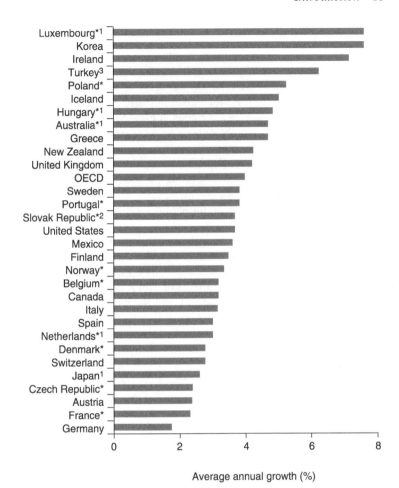

Figure 1.2 Annual Average Growth Rate in Real Health Expenditure Per Capita, 1995–2005

Source: OECD (2007).

appearance. As noted above, population ageing is a further contributor to expenditure growth. The health workforce cannot be overlooked and, with an international shortage of doctors, nurses and other professionals, governments face ongoing pressure to raise remuneration levels and improve working environments (OECD 2008b).

Health system improvement

Despite the increasing expenditure, there is evidence in some countries, particularly the US, that health system performance remains questionable and may even be declining (Commonwealth Fund Commission on a High Performance Health System 2008). In response, various alternatives have been suggested. There have been endeavours in the US, mostly outside of government, to produce plans for a 'high performing health system' that provides universal coverage, equitable access, is affordable (bearing in mind that private insurance is the backbone of US funding), efficient, and protects people from the financial costs of catastrophic illness (for example, Commonwealth Fund 2006; Committee for Economic Development 2007).

Beyond the US, performance improvement includes attempts to increase private sector involvement in public service delivery (see Chapter 7), offering patients 'choice' but also innate incentives for providers to reduce costs and improve efficiency. Efforts also involve setting health system goals and targets, and increased application of methods that restrict access to services and new technologies, drugs and therapies. Decentralization of budgets and planning responsibilities to local agencies has also featured. Countries with social insurance have continually sought ways to increase contributions, reduce coverage, increase efficiency and boost competition in order to drive better system performance (Gauld et al. 2006; Hassenteufel and Palier 2007).

There is considerable international support for the notion that health systems can be improved with attention to services coordination or 'integration' as it is often termed. This is partly in response to the fact that neoliberal arrangements, particularly managerialism, decentralization and contracting, perpetuated gaps between service providers that are typical of health care delivery systems. In other words, they did little to ensure that services, such as primary and secondary care, or public and private providers, were linked. Where competition resulted in a failure to promote sharing of information across systems this has led to duplication of services such as laboratory tests and collection of basic patient information. Despite the rhetoric of being customer focused, neoliberal era arrangements also failed to be patient centred. They were overly oriented toward improving management systems and accountability, with little regard for the patient experience.

In response, it is strongly argued today – from organizations such as the OECD, through to national government policy makers – that health systems ought to be patient centred (Hofmarcher et al. 2007). Funding and organizational models should be aimed at fusing links between, or 'integrating', the various service providers. In contrast with the 'hands-off' approach of neoliberalism, integration naturally requires proactive involvement of management and service providers in the building of coordinated care systems. Integrated care programmes are often developed around specific services such as care for the elderly or treatment of diabetes. They may involve all providers that come in contact with patients from primary care providers through to hospital specialists. Key aims include ensuring that services are carefully coordinated, that the patient experience is 'seamless' and that services are delivered by an appropriate provider. For example, that primary medical care is provided by a community-based practitioner not a hospital specialist. There is considerable anticipation that health information technology will facilitate service integration (see Chapter 4). Britain's Health Action Zones are also an example of integrated service delivery, with a range of different providers working together to improve health outcomes (see Chapter 6).

Of course, there are important arguments that robust primary care can play a central role in developing coordinated services. International agencies such as WHO have renewed calls for emphasizing primary care within health systems (World Health Organization 2008). Research shows that primary care does play an important role, both in terms of improved health system performance as well as in service coordination (Starfield et al. 2005), and several countries have implemented primary care reforms (Saltman et al. 2006). Underpinning these have been the idea that primary and family care should provide the 'gateway' into the health system. Such services should be community based, with patient involvement in planning and governance, should feature a range of providers including general practitioners, and should closely manage the health of their patients (World Health Organization 2008).

Clinical governance (see Chapter 5), which has seen a revitalization of the role of health professionals (as opposed to generic managers of the neoliberal era) in the leadership of provider organizations, has also been commonly cited as pivotal to health system improvement. In part, this has been driven by demands for clinical service quality improvements and renewed regulatory systems. Some countries have pursued arrangements in which primary care services carry the budget for secondary hospital care and other services for formally-enrolled patients, with clinicians responsible for budgetary and service planning on behalf of these patients. In this way, budgetary responsibility is decentralized, but patients will also have a 'medical home' from which their care is coordinated. There will also be an incentive for primary care providers to proactively manage patient health to reduce the likelihood of costly hospitalization. Such trends have been coupled with growing demands for increased patient involvement in governance structures.

Service quality

Since the 1990s across the developed world the quality of health care has received increasing attention (see Chapter 3). This has been largely due to high-profile studies in a range of countries that revealed that medical error, ill-attention to process, and poor communication and coordination within hospitals are responsible for a signficant proportion of hospital patient admissions and deaths (for example Brennan et al. 1991). The focus on quality has also been due to recognition of considerable variation in the practices of individual health practitioners, such as hospital specialists or general practitioners. Variations mean that patients are likely to receive quite different diagnoses, care plans and prescribed medicines from different doctors. The sources of error and variation are often simple, such as incorrectly prescribed medicines, surgical mistakes or inadequate performance monitoring and regulation. However, studies of errors and various government reports have highlighted that mistakes frequently occur as a result of failures within the systems that health professionals work. Again, this has highlighted a need for proactive and hands-on involvement of management, professionals and patients in the crafting of quality improvement programmes.

Of course, practices that endanger and kill patients are of concern to the general public as well as politicians, managers and the health professions. This is for reasons of basic patient safety and the financial costs of medical misadventure and substandard organization. The approach to dealing with quality issues has generally been to bolster the regulation and oversight of health professionals, to improve systems of organization and communication, and to disclose data on individual hospital and practitioner quality and adverse outcomes in the hope that public scrutiny will improve performances. There have also been calls for standardization of medical practice to reduce treatment variations. Medical misadventure, the concentration on quality, and a range of other factors such as the increasing focus on people as consumers and lay access to information via the internet and other sources, has led to a gradual erosion of medical power. It has also led to a growing emphasis on involving the public in health care planning and decision making. Health care providers today are routinely concerned that patient experiences, as measured through exit surveys, complaints and other feedback mechanisms, are positive. This, in turn, creates mounting pressure for improved administrative performance and health professional behaviour, and for better facilities.

The development of systems to monitor quality and provide transparency has also received attention, with elements of managerialism seen in accountability structures but also a quest for data on service standards and quality variations. The application of information technology (Chapter 4) has again been viewed as an important tool for quality improvement.

The drive for quality improvement has led to calls for a range of initiatives. These include health system redesign, with close attention to organizational structures that provide support for high quality clinical practice and delivery of appropriate care (Institute of Medicine 2001). This has naturally created an environment in which health professionals have again become crucial to development, in collaboration with management, of robust patient care systems. It has also created a demand for patient involvement in care planning, for service expansion and for more health spending. The effort to implement funding models that provide incentives for improved performances has been very important. Central to this have been pay for performance and results schemes which reward organizations and health professionals for components of health care delivery. Such schemes can include payments for the percentage of patients screened or vaccinated, who receive appropriate care and are satisfied, the rate of error and hospital readmission, and for the use of information technology in clinical practice (Rosenthal et al. 2004; Rosenthal et al. 2006; Heath et al. 2007). While they can produce positive improvements, as with any system of performance indicators and incentives, performance payments carry the risk of failing to deliver improvements in areas not subject to measurement.

New diseases and health risks

The world is experiencing an increasing incidence of non-communicable diseases including heart and respiratory disease, cancers and diabetes. Heart disease, the biggest single killer, is now responsible for some 30 per cent of global deaths (World Health Organization 2007). Non-communicable diseases are the key cause of death across the developed world. In addition, the prevalence of conditions such as obesity has grown at an alarming rate, virtually doubling in many countries since the 1980s. In 2005, across the OECD countries some 14.6 per cent of people were obese. However, prevalence differs starkly between countries. In the United States and Mexico over 30 per cent were obese. Britain, Greece, Australia and New Zealand all had rates over 20 per cent. Countries with less than 10 per cent incidence of obesity included France, Norway and Switzerland, with Japan and South Korea around 3 per cent (OECD 2007). A concern is that type-2 diabetes, a contributor to which is thought to be obesity, is also on the increase. Diabetes is expensive to treat and associated with other costly health conditions (World Health Organization 2005).

The various non-communicable diseases are related to a range of factors. These include changing lifestyles, behaviour and consumption patterns as well as environmental conditions such as stress levels, the urban environment and access to clean air (see Chapter 6). For health planners and governments alike, non-communicable diseases mean a growing emphasis on changing population behaviour to reduce the risk of such diseases while also developing appropriate support services. They also mean changing the conditions and environments in which people live.

A primary concern of researchers and governments in many developed countries today is growing evidence of inequalities in both access to health services and in health outcomes. These inequalities, which are economic, social and cultural, mean that some people live much longer and healthier lives than others (Wilkinson 2005). For many governments, particularly those of a social democratic persuasion, the inequalities are unjustifiable, unacceptable and, with appropriate policies and actions, reduceable. This means that policy makers and service providers are being required to develop strategies and programmes designed to improve service access for the less well off and marginalized and, ultimately, focus on improving their health. It also means that governments are concentrating more generally on the broader determinants of health in their aim to reduce inequalities. This may include improving the economic circumstances of certain groups, as well as their access to and the quality of welfare, education and housing. It may additionally involve health impact assessments to ensure that public policies will not undermine community health or increase inequalities.

The appearance of new communicable diseases such as Avian Flu, SARS and HIV/AIDS has created a further set of challenges for national and international policy makers. They have produced a need for increased disease surveillance and border control, for analysis of transmission patterns and for health promotion, and for increased capacity to provide treatment services and drugs. They have also posed international governance challenges and focused the attention of national governments on public health (Fidler 2004).

Conclusion

In summary, the post-reform era has seen the emergence of a new health policy agenda in which governments are taking a proactive response to the issues outlined above. The era is characterized by a series of underlying assumptions:

- that policy makers and planners take a hands-on approach in developing programmes designed to better coordinate services, improve quality and efficiency, and change people's behaviour in order to advance their health;
- that health professionals will be central to service governance and decision making;
- that services will be democratized, with the public being encouraged to contribute to decision making; and
- that governments will use a range of mechanisms to achieve policy goals, including public institutions as well as market incentives and the private sector.

This contrasts with, but also draws on elements of, the neoliberal era where it was assumed that the 'market' by itself, combined with various performance incentives and structures such as the purchaser-provider split, would improve service delivery.

BOOK OVERVIEW

This book is designed to help readers learn about a series of policy issues central to the 'new health policy' agenda of developed world governments. It is also aimed at analysis of the impact of the influences outlined in the preceding sections of this chapter, along with the types of emerging organizational forms. Each of the core chapters that follows opens with a list of learning objectives and an introductory overview. Each chapter reviews key developments, arguments and research in the area in question and includes examples of policies in action, largely from Britain, New Zealand and the US. A series of revision questions following the conclusion section is intended to invoke analysis of issues covered in each chapter.

Chapter overview

The funding and organization of health care is the focus of Chapter 2. The chapter overviews the main ways health care is funded. It then considers the different organizational forms found in health systems today where policy makers are seeking population health improvements, service coordination and to boost public participation in decision making and planning, but where there is also a desire to increase accountability, efficiency and, in some cases, competition and the role of the private sector. Such influences are then explored through the experiences of Britain, New Zealand and the US.

Chapter 3 discusses quality and safety issues. It outlines the difficulties of defining what 'quality' is, and why quality and safety are important to the new health policy agenda. The chapter discusses the main sources of quality and safety problems, followed by a review of approaches to quality improvement including 'shame and blame' and 'continuous quality improvement'. Finally, the chapter looks at quality and safety initiatives in practice in Britain, New Zealand and the US.

Information and communications technology (ICT) is the subject of Chapter 4. The chapter looks at the role of information in health care. It discusses the different ways ICT is being applied in health care settings. This includes electronic patient records, management and service support systems. ICT is also empowering patients through the advent of email and the Internet. The chapter notes that governments around the world anticipate that ICT will transform health care, including quality and service coordination and efficiency improvements. The chapter then looks at the high-level strategies introduced by several developed world governments aimed at driving ICT application forward. To illustrate this, the examples of Britain, New Zealand and the US are overviewed.

In Chapter 5, the notion of patient empowerment is further explored. The chapter considers governance, professionalism and public participation. These three themes have been central to debates around how to improve service organization and standards. The chapter looks at what 'governance' is, and then at the idea of 'clinical governance' which many policy makers and health care professionals assert is key to performance improvement. The trends discussed in the chapter have implications for 'professionalism'. Quality and safety issues discussed in Chapter 3 have challenged traditional professional power and prompted the development of 'new professionalism'. This, in turn, has involved the public in the governance of professionals. Governments have also been seeking public and patient involvement in other aspects of their health systems, which is the final focal point of the chapter. As Britain has spearheaded developments overviewed in the chapter, it plays a prominent role in discussions.

As discussed earlier in this chapter, public health issues are high on today's health policy agenda and so Chapter 6 is dedicated to the topic. The chapter notes that public health is often overshadowed by personal health services such as hospital care. It is also influenced by the views of policy makers, such as whether poor health and the alleviation of contributing factors are deemed to be the responsibility of individuals or the state. To illustrate this, the chapter includes a brief history of public health ideas and practice. It then looks at public health issues that are central to the new health policy including globalization and its impacts, health inequalities and social determinants of health, and chronic disease.

Chapter 7, the last of the core chapters, considers the role of the private sector in health systems. The chapter analyses whether the private sector is likely to bring benefits to governments seeking to enhance its role in publicly-funded health care systems. It notes that most health systems feature considerable private sector involvement in an array of different forms, including as a funder and service provider, supplier of pharmaceuticals, and as a partner with the public sector. The chapter lastly looks at the reintroduction of policies designed to inject 'competition and choice' into health systems with a particular emphasis on the British experience as, again, it has been at the forefront of such developments.

Chapter 8 concludes the book, highlighting key themes and lessons from the core subject chapters. It discusses the extent to which neoliberalism and social democracy have influenced each of the policy areas covered in the core subject chapters, and looks at how the intersection of these two philosophical positions might be explained. The conclusion also considers the emerging organizational patterns, as well how the new health policy agenda might be further researched.

2

HEALTH SECTOR FUNDING AND ORGANIZATION

This chapter explores:

- Methods for funding health care
- Funding and organizational reforms in different health systems

INTRODUCTION

Attempts to improve health care delivery and outcomes inevitably revolve around adjustments to the methods of health care funding and to the way in which services are organized. Indeed, the neoliberal health care 'reform' movement of the 1980s and 1990s, which has been widely studied and written about, was predominantly focused on redesigning funding and organizational systems (Ham 1997; Altenstetter and Bjorkman 1997; Ranade 1998; Callahan and Wasunna 2006).

Despite the descent of neoliberalism through the latter part of the 1990s, the quest for health system reform has continued. There have been various reasons for this, as noted in Chapter 1, including that if performance and efficiency can be improved this will result in savings. Even if small, such savings can be significant in the light of the substantial amounts of money that countries spend on health services (the OECD average is around 9 per cent of GDP and the state dominates health spending in most developed countries, with the exception of the US and some East Asian jurisdictions such as Singapore and South Korea).

With this financial focus, many of today's health reform efforts – including pay for performance funding schemes and renewed efforts to induce competition and private sector delivery of public services – look as though they may have been based on neoliberal precepts. Current reforms have also aimed at reorienting health systems to focus on primary care and population health, service integration and quality improvement, as well as on involving the public in service planning and giving them greater choice when it comes to service provision. Such concepts in combination make for complexity and lead to a range of questions. For instance, are policy makers aiming to improve services in the spirit of public service, or to infuse them with market ideals of choice and competition; or are they seeking a bit of both? What sorts of funding and organizational arrangements are different governments pursuing and are they likely to achieve their goals?

This chapter looks at the changing structures for health care funding and organization in developed world countries. First, for the uninitiated, it provides a general overview of the different methods for health care funding. The chapter then outlines how funding and organization have evolved in the health systems of Britain, New Zealand and the US.

HEALTH CARE FUNDING MODELS

In essence, there are three ways in which health care is paid for: through taxes, by social insurance and privately. This section discusses each in turn. Most health systems feature a mix of funding types and sources including government and private. The variations are often in terms of emphasis. For example, the political traditions in some countries will mean a preference for tax funding and higher levels of government than private funding.

Tax funding

Most health systems feature funding from the general tax pool. Countries that favour private funding sources, such as the US, still have a tax component. Health systems where taxation is the primary source of funding include Britain, Canada, Denmark, Spain and New Zealand.

Taxes may be generated from individuals' pay packets or from transactions such as on goods and services. Taxes may also be levied at the national government level, or by local or state government. In countries with federal political systems, such as Australia, Canada and the US, the existence of federal and state taxes goes hand in hand with funding responsibilities. This invariably leads to arguments between federal and state-level governments over responsibility for funding health services. Some countries, such as Australia, have created hypothecated taxes, which are specifically dedicated to health care. This has the potential advantage of showing citizens how much of their tax is being allocated to health care although in the Australian case such tax is only a small portion of the total taxation earmarked for health and it is only applied to those on high incomes. There is also no legal requirement that Australia's government spends its hypothecated health tax on health care (Duckett 2005).

The advantage of tax funding is that it is straightforward to administer and under the control of central government. Political leaders can simply decide how much to spend on health care, increasing this in one year and reducing it in another. In this regard, tax funding may be responsive to public need and demands. However, this is also a potential disadvantage in that there is a lack of transparency. In such situations, neoliberals have long suggested that political lobbying of politicians, along with vote seeking by politicians, leads to inappropriate policy as well as to distortions in the economy to the advantage of certain well-organized interest groups (Olson 1965; Mitchell and Simmons 1994). In response, many countries have sought more transparent methods for allocating funding (which may be deployed within tax based, social insurance or private funding systems). These include distributing funds based on the characteristics of populations served by health care providers, with adjustments for differences in demographics, ethnic composition, and disease prevalence (often called population-based funding). Similarly, diagnostic related group methods, introduced in Chapter 1, aim for cost control as well as equitable allocation among providers, as do uniform fee payment schedules. Pay for performance schemes, meanwhile, reward for achievement of standard expectations.

There is a tendency within predominantly tax funded health systems for public dominance in service delivery. This may be for ideological or historical reasons as with the British NHS. However, it is not uncommon for tax funds to be allocated directly to private providers such as primary care general practitioners or certain private specialties that the public sector is unable to meet the full demand for, as discussed in Chapter 7. In such cases, government may contract with private providers for public service delivery. Government may also be wanting to boost private capacity in order to build a stronger role for the private sector within the health system.

Social insurance

Social insurance is common in many West European countries such as Germany, France and Switzerland (Saltman et al. 2004). It is also found elsewhere, for instance, in Japan, South Korea and Taiwan (Gauld 2005a). Social insurance is government-mandated and therefore compulsory. Funds are risk-pooled and collected from a combination of salaries and employer contributions the levels of which are set by government. Following its title, social insurance is not risk related and so there is the capacity for delivering on goals of equity. The administration of social insurance funds varies. In some health systems, this is the responsibility of a single national agency, as in Taiwan and South Korea (Lee et al. 2008). This agency may be under the close control of government, or operate with some independence under statute. Single bodies mean that funds administration and the implementation of government policy are both simple, but for the public they offer no choice and could lack incentives to improve performance.

Other health systems feature multiple social insurers as in Germany, France and Japan. These may be designed to serve specific geographic areas or groups of people. In Japan, for example, there are different 'tiers' of insurance, each with multiple providers, for public servants and employees of large companies, for small business employees, and for those of less means. The government subsidizes the tiers that provide for the less well off to ensure affordability and insurer viability (Ikegami 2005). Such subsidies are commonplace in social insurance systems as governments need to ensure that the unemployed, elderly and indigent have health care coverage. In some countries, such as Germany and the Netherlands, there have been attempts to induce competition among insurers by allowing people to move between providers. Yet this has been complex as providers are prohibited from denying coverage to any applicant (Mossialos and Dixon 2002: 19).

In general, social insurance is combined with a schedule of fees paid for treatment services based on claims made by providers. This schedule may need to be managed by the government or an agency on its behalf and renegotiated periodically to reflect service costs. Social insurance generally funds a significant portion of costs, meaning that patients will have to pay part of this on delivery of service. Co-payment or out-of-pocket expenditure differs between countries. South Korea, for instance, requires that patients pay around 40 per cent of costs not covered by social insurance. In Western Europe out-of-pocket payments, which may include co-payments as well as expenditure on health care that is not subsidized by social insurance, differ between countries from as much as 33 per cent in Switzerland to around 7 per cent in Luxembourg (Figueras et al. 2004: 113).

Advantages of social insurance include transparency in that public reporting reveals the nature of expenditure and resource allocation and shows where funds are failing to meet with the number of claims made. In this way, social insurance may provide a clear justification to the public for increased levies (or taxes as these may be perceived by the public). Distance from political leaders is also often viewed as an advantage especially in countries where there is low public trust in politicians. A potential disadvantage is that multiple insurers can mean complex administration and reduced capacity for delivering equitably. Rising costs can also prove politically difficult. These generally are passed directly on to the public by way of increased premiums. However, substantial increases may create pressure for the government to top-up insurance funds from the general tax pool or search for ways to limit the range of services eligible to be funded by social insurance.

Private funding

Private funding may be used to pay for both public and private services. Private providers, of course, will generally charge full cost for their services. In some cases, government may be a purchaser of these and therefore fully fund eligible patients, or be a subsidizer and require that patients share some of the costs. Public providers may also operate on such a cost-sharing model.

Private funding comes from a variety of sources including out-of-pocket payments for services provided. Such payments are common for general practitioner services in countries such as Australia, Canada and New Zealand. Cost-sharing also occurs where private (or social) insurance pays part of the bill, but requires that patients contribute. In the US, insurance arrangements routinely include a 'deductible' which is the amount that patients are required to pay in a year (perhaps $1000.00) before insurance coverage commences. After that, the insured may still be required to pay a portion of the cost of any services provided.

Of course, private insurance is commonplace in many countries, with the role of this depending on the way in which the system functions. In some (characteristically tax-funded) health systems, private insurance is used to fund non-urgent treatments that the recipients might normally have to wait a considerable time for the public sector to provide. Countries such as the US are heavily reliant on private insurance as the predominant funding mechanism (Jonas et al. 2007). Private insurance in the US tends to be paid for by employers who, in turn, offset the costs of this with various government tax breaks.

Medical savings accounts (MSAs) are a form of private funding developed in Singapore, but also in limited use in the US, South Africa and parts of China. MSAs in Singapore are mandatory with workers and employers contributing a percentage of wages into accounts which are the property of individual account holders (Barr 2005). Unlike social or private health insurance, there is no risk pooling (in Singapore only family members can share funds with one another; Asher and Nandy 2006). The incentive is for individuals to pay close attention to the costs of health care as these are drawn from a personal account. MSAs often need to be linked with additional catastrophic insurance due to the lack of risk pooling. This is the case in Singapore where MSAs actually pay only a small portion of total health care costs, with deductables, government subsidies, employer benefits and out-of-pocket payments also contributing.

The perceived advantage of private funding is that it provides incentives to patients to pay attention to the costs of health care and in turn to focus on being healthy as the alternative, being unwell, bears a financial cost. Private funding also is equated with notions of patient choice and determination in that where individuals are responsible for costs they will demand improved services and quality. This said, private funding tends to be inequitable, and even unethical, as services may be denied to those unable to pay. Private insurance usually involves considerable administration and transactions costs (a noteworthy feature of the US health system) due to requirements of risk rating (calculating benefit packages, coverage levels and premiums), billing and claims administration, contracting with providers, and service utilization review (Mossialos and Dixon 2002).

HEALTH SYSTEM REFORMS

This section illustrates the preceding discussions and the contextual material from Chapter 1 by looking at the recent history of health funding and organizational reforms in different health systems. It considers the cases of the tax-funded 'national' systems of Britain and New Zealand, and the private sector market-oriented United States.

Britain and New Zealand

There are many commonalities between Britain and New Zealand. Both are electoral democracies, so political parties and politicians are deeply involved in shaping public policy that accords with their political ideologies. Both have 'national' health systems that are tax-funded. Both also have a recent history of successive reforms to their funding and organizational arrangements influenced by neoliberalism and then social democracy. Their health systems both now feature a web of market structures and incentives, along with social democratic aims.

The British NHS was created in 1946 in the spirit of building a 'national' tax-funded health system intended to provide universal service access – from primary care through to hospital services – to all British citizens. With similar origins and aims, New Zealand created the world's first national health system in 1938. That said, New Zealand has frequently looked to the NHS for policy lessons. In both countries, national health system creation required bargaining with the medical profession, predominantly in private practice. The resulting arrangements remain in place today. That is, of general practice being largely provided by private practitioners, with considerable government subsidies, while the public sector dominates hospital services. Both health systems share a tradition of being centrally administered by a government agency and of health professionals serving in key decision-making posts at the regional planning and hospital level. In 2006, total health expenditure in Britain was 8.4 per cent, against the OECD average of 8.9 per cent. The NHS was responsible for 87 per cent of this expenditure. It is one of the world's largest organizations and employs over one million people from primary care through to hospital specialists. At 9.3 per cent of GDP, New Zealand was above the OECD average for health expenditure, with the public system accounting for just under 80 per cent of the total (OECD 2008a).

Britain

The NHS reforms occurred in the era of Prime Minister Margaret Thatcher (in power from 1979–1990). A review, influenced by economists who criticized the NHS for lacking incentives to improve performace (e.g. Enthoven 1985), suggested the single-payer tax funding system be retained, but that the organization of services be formed into an 'internal market' (Department of Health 1989). Implemented in 1991, the internal market was intended to induce incentives to boost system performance, especially reducing costs, streamlining management and improving quality. The reforms saw the previously integrated roles of funding and managing services within health authorities split. Health authorities were transformed into purchasers, responsible within a government determined budget for negotiating contracts with providers to meet the needs of their respective communities.

New NHS trusts were created to be responsible for management of hospitals and community health services. The trusts remained public organizations within the NHS but subjected to business discipline under the control of new government-appointed management boards. Trust income was largely to be determined in accordance with contracts won from NHS purchasers. In this way, the trusts were to 'compete' with one another.

The performance of the Thatcher reforms was mixed. The internal market shifted the balance of power within the NHS. The introduction of GP fundholding allowed larger general practices to be 'fundholders' for various routine procedures and, thus, purchase services on behalf of their patients from local NHS trusts (Glennester et al. 1993). With trust hospitals dependent on GP fundholders and purchasing health authorities for funding, they proactively sought to market their services. They became less fixated with internal administrative issues and increasingly concerned with satisfying 'customers': their patients, as well as service purchasers. GP fundholding led to practices carefully studying their referral and prescribing patterns and extending their scope of practice. Some fundholders employed additional staff in areas such as physiotherapy, nutrition and counselling. The internal market naturally required considerable administration and regulation to make it work although there was little consistency in the application of rules and wide variations in the levels of competition in different geographical areas (see Smith and Goddard 2000).

The election in 1997 of Tony Blair's New Labour government brought an agenda of further NHS reform, as spelled out in *The New NHS: Modern, Dependable* (Department of Health 1998). Blair's government also stood for a new set of social democratic principles that included substantially increasing government funding for health care, improving service access and quality, collaboration among service providers, and a public health focus. Yet its initial health policies retained elements of the internal market including the purchaser-provider split and decentralization. As such, the system of providers competing for funding contracts remained in place. The primary care arrangements were also retained, but subsequently altered. New Labour appeared keen to distance itself from the internal market, arguing that the 'business' model of health care led to fragmentation, was unfair to patients and inefficient. This is where its policies for integration of services fitted in, as well as the focus on public health improvement.

Key changes included abolishing GP fundholding and replacing this with Primary Care Groups which general practitioners were compulsorily required to join and play a leadership role in. Each group had responsibility for around 100,000 patients and for commissioning (or buying) most of the services for their respective populations. In effect, the Primary Care Groups model meant that patients lost some of their choice among providers as such decisions were made by the group they were enrolled in. In its early years, the Blair government created the National Institute for Health and Clinical Excellence (NICE), aimed to develop guidelines for clinical and cost-effective decision-making, and various other bodies committed to quality and service improvement and performance monitoring. It created a series of National Service Frameworks aimed at achieving national consistency in the delivery of services. A Commission for Health Improvement (now the Healthcare Commission) was established to monitor NHS provider performances against the National Performance Framework, and to inspect service quality and intervene where failures occured (Smith and Goddard 2000).

In 2000, amid charges that the NHS was in a perpetual state of crisis, the government boosted NHS funding which, at 7 per cent of GDP, was below the European and OECD average. An annual funding increase from 2000–08 of 7.5 per cent, more than double the previous yearly injection, was announced along with the 'NHS Plan' for how this would be spent (Department of Health 2000b). A series of clinical (e.g. improve quality, reduce waiting lists and improve service access) and public health (e.g. NHS organizations collaborate with one another to reduce inequalities) targets were produced for this. Hospital organizations were to be given 'star' ratings for their performances. Those with more stars were given greater autonomy over the use of resources and additional discretionary funding (Mannion et al. 2005). The Plan contained provisions for public–private partnerships for building projects, and for use of the private sector to perform public work such as elective surgery. The Plan also focused on improving clinical standards through new systems of professional self-regulation and monitoring. This was combined with a programme to appoint senior health professionals to key national posts in areas such as cancer services and mental health to lead change where 'managers' had been seen to fail. A key area of focus for the new funding, aimed at service improvement, was a new national contract between the NHS and GPs. Very different from the prior funding model, which was a basic payment for each enrolled patient, the new contract was based on pay for performance. GPs would be paid in accordance with adherence to a series of clinical and other indicators (Campbell et al. 2007).

Since around 2002, a range of market mechanisms have been reintroduced into the NHS. There has been a renewed emphasis on decentralization of decision-making to local level managers. In 2003, the government created a new Foundation Trust hospital status awarded to strong performers. Those with Foundation Trust status are given considerable managerial and financial freedom, including the right to raise funds from private investors for capital works. The aim is for all NHS Trusts to eventually have Foundation status. While standard NHS Trusts remain under central government control, the financial performance of Foundation Trusts is regulated by the independent Monitor, established in 2004, and quality by the Healthcare Commission. From 2004, government policy has permitted private providers to contract with the NHS as Independent Sector Treatment Centres. Such centres provide surgery for NHS patients while creating competition among a more diverse range of providers (Pollock and Godden 2008). By 2008, as noted in Chapter 7, independent treatment centres performed 10 per cent of NHS procedures.

There have also been changes to the 'demand' side of care. Primary Care Trusts (PCTs) were created in 2000 to commission services from NHS Trusts. A 2006 reform saw a reduction from 300 to around 150 PCTs. Alongside PCTs, a 'practice-based commissioning' policy has required that some decision-making is devolved to the general practice level. In parallel, the pay for performance policy was deepened by the introduction of payment by results (or procedure performed based on patients seen and case-mix). This is intended to improve efficiency and quality among both private and public providers of NHS services. The final market mechanism, and in keeping with payment by results (or patients seen), was the reintroduction, in 2006, of patient choice. The idea here is that patients with non-urgent conditions be given a choice of five service providers and be provided with information about those providers to aid their decision (Mays 2008).

In 2008, the delivery of the government's so-called 'Darzi report', named after its principal author, surgeon Lord Ara Darzi, spelled out yet another set of directions for the NHS (Department of Health 2008b). Whether major changes will result remains to be seen as, for the most part, the Darzi report reiterated developments already underway. These include focusing the NHS on keeping people well, rather than treating illness; acknowledging the important contribution of clinicians and empowering them to lead NHS change; and localizing NHS planning and decision-making processes. Of course, there have been criticisms that the current directions for the NHS, of ensuring that funding is public and tax-funded, while facilitating patient choice among a range of competing NHS and private providers, may be unlikely to produce more effective or efficient services. As will be discussed in Chapter 7, they may even undermine the viability of some NHS services. Suggested alternatives include developing fully integrated service delivery systems that could compete with one another (Ham 2008).

New Zealand

In a similar pattern to Britain, New Zealand policy was heavily influenced by neoliberal ideas from around 1984–1999. Initially, this was under a Labour government (1984–90), then a conservative National government (1990–99). Concerned about health system performance, especially hospital administration and efficiency, the Labour government commissioned a series of health system reviews. One of these, chaired by a pro-market businessman, suggested market-oriented structures along the lines of the Thatcher internal market reforms (Gibbs et al. 1988). It was not until 1991, under the National government, that these ideas were put into practice. The health system was then radically reformed with purchasing and providing split. Four new Regional Health Authorities were created to undertake purchasing and to contract with any provider – public or private – for the delivery of publicly-funded services. A Public Health Commission was created to purchase public health services (Bandaranayake 1994). Public hospitals were restructured into Crown Health Enterprises, run by managers and executive boards, which were expected to return a dividend to the government on funds received. With competitive contracting for funding, costs were intended to be cut and efficiency improved. There was also an attempt to define a basket of 'core services' so that the purchasers would know exactly what services they were responsible for buying. In primary care, general practitioners, who previously were mostly sole operators, grouped into new Independent Practitioner Associations – with similarities to British GP fundholding groups – to improve their bargaining power with the purchasers.

The reforms were short-lived, with numerous problems. The attempt to define core services failed, so there were no clear limitations on what was being purchased. The Crown Health Enterprises were unable to cut costs or close 'unviable' services and, for the most part, required additional government funding to develop their 'businesses'. Morale among health professionals suffered and there were few private competitors for hospital and other service contracts. This meant Regional Health Authorities simply contracted with existing public providers. A brief attempt at hospital part-charges proved expensive to administer and was very unpopular, producing considerable political discomfort.

On the upside, there were some efficiency gains, information was improved, and the Independent Practitioner Associations revitalized general practice. Like the British situation, there were experiments with fundholding with savings able to be reinvested in additional services. Following the 1996 election, the system was re-reformed. The four purchasers were combined into a single national purchaser. Hospitals were no longer required to return a profit. Instead, they were to focus on 'public service' but also to be 'businesslike'. In line with international trends, there was a shift in emphasis toward reducing inequalities, developing national service standards to reduce variations in elective treatment waiting times and service delivery capacity, and toward service integration. Yet the purchaser-provider split remained at the heart of the system and hospital governance was largely by private sector appointees directed to run hospitals in a 'business-like' manner (Gauld 2001).

In 1999, a re-elected Labour government, which had distanced itself from its romance with neoliberalism in the 1980s, brought further health system reforms (Devlin et al. 2001). Implemented in 2001, these were in keeping with the new government's social democratic orientation and goals of democratizing and decentralizing health care decision-making, reducing inequalities, improving service access particularly for disadvantaged groups, and reorienting the health system toward collaboration and public health improvement.

Getting the reforms in place was, like any reform process, exhaustive for the health sector (Gauld 2003).

New structures included 21 regionally-based District Health Boards (DHBs). Each is funded based on the characteristics of the population they serve and was built around the existing hospital groups. Each has responsibility for planning and funding services from primary through to hospital care for the district's population. The government's preference is for funding public services. Thus, use of the private sector for elective surgery is restricted. Contracting continues to be central to the funding process, but there is limited competition among providers. Instead, the government has chosen to build capacity within the public sector and drive performance with a series of national goals and targets laid out in the New Zealand Health Strategy and other documents (King 2000; Minister of Health 2007). These broadly social democratic goals have been offset by application of neoliberal performance management tools.

DHB performance expectations and service goals are contained in annual contracts and plans and regularly reviewed by the government which keeps a tight reign on DHBs. There are a range of financial and other sanctions on DHB management for poor performance. For example, DHBs that fail to manage within budget will be subject to reduced autonomy and increased central government control. Those failing to deliver elective and other services on target face financial penalties. As such, some DHBs purchase elective services from private providers. Others resort to restricting the number of patients allowed to be placed on waiting lists while 'dumping' those unable to be treated within the government's targeted timeframe of six months. Affected patients have the option of paying privately for treatment, or can attempt to re-enter the public system.

The 21 DHBs each feature a mix of elected and appointed members. They are required to consult the community in their planning and needs assessments and to coordinate services. Despite the rhetoric and new democratic structures, the DHBs remain under firm central government control and must adhere to a range of national policies as set out in their annual contracts. Staff employed by the DHBs, including Chief Executives, are similarly motivated by contractual obligations. Despite substantial funding increases since 1999 (averaging 7–8 per cent per annum), service demand continues to increase and funding remains tight. As such, DHBs are perpetually looking to reduce costs and streamline services, leading to charges among health professionals that this is the primary focus of 'management'. There have long been suggestions that 21 DHBs is too many for a country of 4 million people, especially given the requirements for collaboration and the substantial transaction costs associated with 21 separate funding bodies (Gauld 2005d).

Since 2003, the government has promoted formation of new Primary Health Organizations (PHOs). These capitalize on the organizational efforts of GPs through the 1990s, but require a broader professional base and community orientation. There are presently around eighty PHOs covering 97 per cent of the population. The Ministry of Health initially drove PHO formation but subsequently handed responsibility to District Health Boards who provide PHO funding. Each PHO must have a list of formally-enrolled patients on which capitation funding is calculated (previously GPs simply maintained a patient register and were paid a fee for service). They must also show evidence of a range of primary care provider members, not just GPs, and a non-profit governance structure that includes community representatives. Considerable new funding was made available for PHO formation, providing incentives for this, and also to reduce patient part-charges. Extra funding is also available for 'care plus' initiatives designed for people with chronic disease, for 'services to improve access' and for health promotion (Gauld and Mays 2006). The government, however, has continued to drive PHO performance with a pay for performance scheme, with payments for achievement of various public health and financial objectives (District Health Boards New Zealand 2005).

Despite the succession of reforms to the New Zealand health system, it remains in a state of flux. As discussed in Chapter 3, quality has received limited attention, at least at the national policy level, while pressure is mounting for greater coordination across the DHBs – even DHB mergers – and government leadership in this. Similarly, while primary care has been at the forefront of recent government policy, there is evidence that several primary care policy issues demand attention. These include the large number of PHOs (many with small numbers of patients), how to develop truly multidisciplinary organizations in an environment where funding favours GPs, and whether PHOs should be geographically based or compete with one another (Gauld 2008b).

United States

Public policy in the US reflects a set of quintessentially American 'values' of freedom, individualism and individual rights, small government (and even an aversion to government involvement in society, or to government-led policy change), and a preference for private service provision (Blank and Burau 2004: 46–7; Callahan and Wasunna 2006; Jonas et al. 2007). The federal political system in the US – with an elected Senate and House of Representatives, and Presidential right to veto any policy once it has been approved by the two houses – is notable for the fact that it is designed to make it difficult to achieve policy change. Perhaps not surprisingly, the large-scale changes implemented in Britain and New Zealand simply do not occur in the US. Changes tend to be incremental and often at the individual state level but, since the early 1990s, pressure for more fundamental change has been mounting.

At 15.3 per cent of GDP, the US spends more than any other country in the world on health care (OECD 2008a). Per capita spending is around 50 per cent above the next biggest spenders in the OECD, and over double the OECD average. Yet some 47 million Americans do not have health insurance. As such, they lack guaranteed access to health care and often face astronomical personal costs as a result. The US has what is often considered to be a 'private' health system featuring a complex mix of private and public arrangements. It is sometimes suggested of the US that the term 'system', which connotes organization and logic, is misleading (Oberlander 2002). Health policy today in the US is poised at a juncture between embracing of neoliberal market concepts for organization, with mounting pressure – spurred on by the election of President Obama in 2008 – for pursuit of social democratic goals.

Health insurance is at the heart of private arrangements (accounting for around 55 per cent of total health expenditure), with most people receiving insurance coverage via their employer. Thus, employment and employers offering good insurance is important to employees. Employers, in turn, buy coverage from any number of private insurance providers. These organizations then purchase services from specific specialists, hospitals and primary care physicians. Despite the rhetoric of choice as fundamental to US health care, for many Americans choice is limited. This is because employees must simply accept insurance packages that their employers have subscribed to. That said, depending on the plan, the insured often have considerable choice among primary care physicians, specialists and hospital services. In some cases, such as California's Kaiser Permanente, which covers 8.5 million people, the insurer is fully integrated and runs its own 'health system' (Feachem et al. 2002). Most insurance packages feature a deductible, and also require co-payments at point of service. Such costs will vary from plan to plan. A cheaper plan, for example, may feature higher co-payments and deductables.

Much of the 45 per cent of public expenditure is channelled through the Medicaid and Medicare schemes which, respectively, provide government-funded (a combination of Federal and State) insurance for the less well off and the elderly. Those not covered by private or public insurance may be out of work, unable to afford insurance (self-employed, for instance), or in employment that does not provide coverage. Increasing evidence shows that the expanding costs of insurance, reflecting health care cost increases, is resulting in growing numbers of previously insured people going without cover or being underinsured. The high cost of health care to individuals and lack of insurance to pay for required care is one of the leading causes of bankruptcy in the US (Himmelstein and Woolhandler 2001: 24–5; Himmelstein et al. 2005). The US is also notable for stark inequalities in service delivery and health outcomes (Ayanian et al. 2000) and for only delivering around 55 per cent of indicated care to patients (McGlynn et al. 2003).

There have been periodic attempts to create a national health insurance scheme. The most recent was President Bill Clinton's 'health security' plan. This aimed to create universal insurance coverage by requiring all employers to provide insurance to their workers, and by providing subsidies to small businesses and the unemployed to purchase their own insurance. Opposition to the plan, largely to the idea that government would preside over changes to the status quo, which served many quarters well (e.g. businesses and individuals happy with *their* insurance arrangements), led to its defeat in 1994 (Oberlander 2002). In its wake, and on the tail of cost growth pressure, the 'managed care' movement grew (Dudley and Luft 2001).

Managed care refers to arrangements designed to limit the costs of individual health encounters. It stems from early experiments with groups of providers working together to provide services under pre-specified rules around how much would be paid for particular services. In this way, managed care differs from the traditional fee for service model where providers simply submitted a claim for services delivered. Thus, managed care aims to both restrict the range of providers a patient might have access to, but also control the costs for an insurer. Many managed care variants emerged, including pre-paid capitation models. While spending growth initially slowed as managed care expanded, it gained pace again from the start of the new millennium (Oberlander 2002). Moreover, from the late 1990s a 'backlash' against managed care emerged, driven by concerns that the focus of insurers on cost control had undermined service quality and led to unwarranted service denials (Blendon et al. 1998). This, combined with the growing numbers of uninsured and ever-increasing growth in expenditure, has fuelled calls for reform.

There have been many other initiatives and pressures for change. As noted in Chapter 3, quality has been high on the agenda since at least the release of the Institute of Medicine report, *To Err is Human* (Institute of Medicine 2000). Information technology was at the centre of President George W. Bush's agenda (see Chapter 4), with high hopes that this will produce cost reductions, improved quality and patient-centred care. Considerable effort is required to increase the utilization of information technology in the US health system, which remains low by international standards. In addition, many high-profile non-government and private organizations have undertaken research into the health system, highlighting the need for change and producing blueprints for reform.

In 2006, for instance, the Commonwealth Fund issued a high-profile 'scorecard' for a high performing health system highlighting quality, equity, efficiency and access deficiencies (Commonwealth Fund Commission on a High Performance Health System 2006). An updated scorecard, released in 2008, showed that, despite increased health care expenditure, performance had declined (Commonwealth Fund Commission on a High Performance Health System 2008). The Fund has continued to advocate for health care coverage improvements and reforms that would inevitably involve a larger role for government. In 2007, the Committee for Economic Development, which represents major business and economic interests, unveiled its plan for a reformed and expanded insurance system (Committee for Economic Development 2007). The Committee noted that, since 2000, health care costs for employers have increased at five times the rate of inflation and that, due to cost, employers are progressively pulling out of providing health insurance for employees. Small business employees, in particular, are increasingly being denied health insurance. The Committee's recommendation was that government should provide a 'fixed-dollar credit' to individuals that would enable them to choose among competing insurance plans. These plans would be accessible via a series of government-created but independent regional 'insurance exchanges' that provide a single entry point for those seeking insurance (Committee for Economic Development 2007).

There appears to be growing acceptance among US politicians

and the general public that health care ought to be more universally accessible and affordable. Reflecting this, some US states have been working to create universal insurance coverage. Generally, state initiatives have involved bi-partisan approaches that bring together federal, state and private insurers to extend insurance subsidies, build low-cost plans with limited but essential coverage, and drive down service delivery prices. In Massachusetts, larger employers who fail to provide insurance are subject to financial penalties, while an insurance exchange has been established to provide information about competing plans to those seeking coverage. Tennessee's CoverTN scheme, designed for those on low incomes, is focused on providing primary medical care and outpatient services, access to a range of generic medicines, and limited hospital care, with a ceiling on claims able to be made within any one year. The state government in Louisiana is steering low-income Medicare beneficiaries into private health care plans, intended to reduce costs and improve service quality, that the government pays a fixed per-patient amount to. Physicians and hospitals will, in turn, be paid for outcomes with incentives for good performance, instead of the prior system which compensated for volume of visits and procedures. Health care was a core theme in campaigning for the US Presidential election of 2008 with both the Democratic and Republican candidates arguing for expanded health care insurance coverage and an increased federal and state government role in this. Health care remains high on President Barack Obama's agenda, with the likelihood of reform growing with an important coalition of businesses, politicians from both political parties, and public interest groups all recognizing that change is needed.

However, at the heart of proposals remains the emphasis on private arrangements and competing plans raising questions over whether universal coverage can ever be achieved. Another challenge for the US, as noted, is improving the overall performance of the system to ensure that all North Americans, not just those with good insurance, are able to access and receive high quality care. US health care remains dominated by expensive specialist and hospital services. A 2008 study reported that primary care was unattractive to medical graduates (National Association of Community Health Centers 2008). Most primary care practitioners are licensed specialists such as pediatricians (who provide child primary care consultations), internal medicine graduates (adult consultations), and gynaecologists (serving as womens' GPs). Finally, the organization of health care in the US remains fragmented, with the exception of systems such as

Kaiser, discussed above, and the Veterans Health Administration (Oliver 2008). This is a consequence of competition and government inability to coordinate, or even demand coordination, across such a large and diverse system, but also the aversion to government intervention.

CONCLUSION

This chapter outlined the different ways health care is funded. Against this background, and the contextual material laid out in Chapter 1, health system reforms in Britain, New Zealand and the US were then overviewed. Two questions were posed at the outset of the chapter. These were around the health policy strategies being developed by governments; and whether the structures being pursued are likely to facilitate achievement of these strategies.

As illustrated in the chapter, Britain and New Zealand appear to be pursuing complex and sometimes conflicting combinations of both market and social democratic oriented policy arrangements. Perhaps as a consequence of this, the organizational forms that have developed are similarly complicated. Where Britain and New Zealand diverge is in the way their policy mix has been developed. In Britain, neoliberal arrangements are aimed at driving improved performance, especially by promoting competitive behaviour among public and private providers. The intended outcome is to deliver on social democratic goals such as expanding service access and improving quality. In New Zealand, where local decision-making, provider collaboration and public participation are key aims, neoliberal concepts are being applied to funding arrangements including performance incentives and contracting between funders and providers. Neoliberal influences are naturally evident in the market-oriented US. However, there is mounting pressure for reforms aimed at creating universal and affordable service access and for government involvement in this. As with Britain and New Zealand, concerns about health care quality, primary care and inequality are also on the policy agenda.

Whether the structures in place can achieve each of the country's goals is questionable. As Chapter 7 discusses, there is little evidence to suggest that competition and increased private sector involvement in health systems improves service efficiency or quality. The US is a profound example of this although, as noted, components of its system perform well. Britain's path therefore could be a difficult (even an incorrect) one, yet one in which, following the Darzi report, health care professionals will be handed increasing responsibility for leading. Moreover, there is mounting evidence that ongoing health system reform can be damaging, with New Zealand's experience a case in point. Despite successive restructurings, its system remains troubled.

The diffused nature of health care organization in the US, with private market dominance, means it is difficult to determine its policy goals, and that these would correspondingly be problematic to achieve. The goal of expanding insurance coverage is an illustrative example. The Federal government has restricted capacity to simply increase tax funding for health care coverage, as Britain and New Zealand can do with relative ease. Instead, it must work with industry and the federal Medicare and Medicaid schemes and promote state-level initiatives. The US faces similar challenges with regard to issues such as primary care and information technology development, and with quality improvement. The latter is the subject of the next chapter.

QUESTIONS FOR FURTHER DISCUSSION

1. What are the advantages and disadvantages of the different models of health care funding?
2. How does the funding of health care differ between Britain, New Zealand and the US?
3. How does the organization of health care differ between Britain, New Zealand and the US?
4. Reconsidering the reforms within the three health systems outlined in the last sections of the chapter, was there evidence of neoliberalism, social democracy, or a combination of both driving policy?

HEALTH CARE QUALITY AND SAFETY

This chapter explores:

- The differing dimensions of quality
- Where concerns about quality and safety come from
- The main reasons why quality and safety problems occur
- Approaches to improving quality in different health systems

INTRODUCTION

A core concern of policy makers today, particularly across the developed world, is with the quality of health care. Essentially, quality refers to the capacity for health care professionals, the organizations and structures they work within, and for health systems per se to provide services that are delivered in a consistent manner and that do not pose a threat to patients' safety and lives. Concerns about quality have been driven by a series of studies that provided evidence that patients are often at risk within health care settings as a consequence of inadequate quality control. These studies show that patients have unacceptably high rates of complications and deaths as a result. Quality problems are also responsible for high rates of hospital readmission.

Further highlighting the demand for quality improvement and for assurances that services are safe have been high profile cases of criminal activity and negligence by medical professionals that have gone unchecked. Examples include the cases of Harold Shipman and of the Bristol Hospital Inquiry in the United Kingdom. Of course, quality problems not only affect patients, often terribly so; they also pose considerable costs for health service providers and health systems. Despite the efforts of governments and provider organizations, and a proliferation of research into quality, the problems remain. The solutions hinge on different theories about how to improve quality and are often piecemeal and difficult to apply. The reasons for this are the inherent complexity of health care and fact that it is often not individuals but the systems within which they deliver services that are to blame for quality lapses.

As discussed in this chapter, one set of approaches to quality improvement involves use of market-type mechanisms and increased control over clinical work and might therefore be seen as emerging from a neoliberal position. Other approaches, employed in combination with new regulation and governance structures, align more closely with social democratic ideals. The picture as such is one of complexity.

This chapter overviews key issues in health care quality and safety. It opens with a brief discussion of the concept of quality. Next, it looks at the rise of concerns about quality, the main sources of quality problems and the different strategies to remedy these including 'shame and blame' and 'continuous quality improvement' approaches. Third, the chapter looks at quality improvement efforts in Britain, New Zealand and the United States. The conclusion revisits two questions: how does the mix of quality improvement initiatives in the three countries compare; and are current efforts to improve quality and safety adequate?

DEFINING HEALTH CARE QUALITY

The fact that defining health care quality is not a straightforward exercise is indicative of the difficulties that those attempting to improve quality can face. While aspects of quality are able to be measured (for example, how many patients per thousand receive the wrong medicines), quality is often a subjective issue (how do patients feel about a service, and how might our system be improved?). Its definition, therefore, depends on the perspectives of those doing the defining – whether it is medical professionals, managers, funders, politicians or patients. For patients, quality may be more about whether there are treatment delays, about the bedside manner of doctors, and the extent to which there are varying messages coming from different health professionals. Managers and policy makers may be focused on issues such as reducing the costs related to medical errors that compromise patient health, or on creating conditions that allow for practitioners to pay attention to the quality of care they provide. Health professionals, for their part, may see quality as a process of ensuring that they routinely provide the right diagnosis and treatments, based on the most up-to-date medical knowledge. Obviously, with these different players involved, quality applies to literally all components of the health system. This can make the task of working out how to improve quality perplexing. It also means that there are multiple possibilities for quality improvement. Resulting policies, of course, will also be contingent on the preferences of policy makers. Some may prefer incentive-based systems aimed at boosting performance through competition and control. Others will opt for collaborative approaches to system or service improvement.

Reflecting the above, researchers and policy makers have often suggested that quality has various dimensions. These, in turn, provide a focus for policy development and action. An example of this is the list produced by the United States Institute of Medicine, which has produced some high profile reports that have placed quality firmly on the policy agenda in that country (Institute of Medicine 2000; 2001). The Institute of Medicine (2000) suggests that a quality health service should be focused on:

- safety and the avoidance of patient injuries;
- being patient centred, respecting and responsive to individual preferences, needs and values;
- timeliness, concerned with reducing delays and ensuring access to care;
- equity, in that all people should receive the same quality of care regardless of gender, ethnicity, geographic location or ability to pay;
- effectiveness, ensuring that service delivery is based on sound scientific knowledge, avoiding overuse of ineffective therapies, underuse of ineffective therapies and misuse of therapies;
- efficiency, making the best use of services and avoiding waste.

The Institute of Medicine's list is a not uncommon approach. Indeed, several of the developed world's governments have produced similar frameworks but the factors included tend to differ among them in keeping with the issues that policy makers have decided should be emphasized. One government, for example, may highlight the need to be patient centred and improve clinical processes; another may also seek to make information about quality publicly available so that patients can be fully informed about the potential risks from different service providers.

THE RISE OF QUALITY AND SAFETY CONCERNS

Service quality and safety are quite possibly among the most crucial issues facing the developed world's health systems today, and with good reason. But this has not always been the case. Indeed, quality was not really a concern for policy makers or health professionals until various studies revealed it to be an issue. It was simply assumed that good quality physicians and other health care providers were produced by ensuring high standards in medical and other training schools.

The results from the first of a series of groundbreaking quality studies, the Harvard Medical Practice Study, appeared in 1991 (Brennan et al. 1991). The researchers behind this study sought to identify adverse events (injuries caused by medical error) by scrutinizing the medical records of some 30,000 patients in New York State. Adverse events were defined as any incident that resulted in prolonged hospitalization or produced a disability at the time of hospital discharge. The study found that 3.7 per cent of hospital patients were victims of an adverse event. Of these, 2.6 per cent suffered a permanent injury, and 13.6 per cent died. The Harvard study was subsequently replicated, with a 2.9 per cent adverse event rate found (Thomas et al. 2000).

Similar studies in Australia and New Zealand identified adverse events in 16.6 and 12.9 per cent of hospitalized patients respectively (Wilson et al. 1995; Davis et al. 2002). Meanwhile, a British government study found that around 11.7 per cent of patients were at risk of adverse events (Vincent et al. 2001). However, these studies used wider definitions of adverse events than the American studies. In the Australian and British cases, around half of the adverse events were unpreventable. An example of this is a terminally ill patient requiring emergency life saving medicine that the patient then reacts to and dies from.

The impact of the adverse event studies is much greater when translated into sheer numbers of people affected. Not until the 1999 release of the Institute of Medicine's report, *To Err is Human*, did the American public and its political leaders realize the extent to which hospitals were dangerous and medical care prone to quality failures. Based on calculations from the Harvard studies, the

Institute's report suggested that at least 44,000 and perhaps as many as 98,000 North Americans die each year as a result of preventable errors when in hospital care, at a cost to the country of between US$17 billion and $29 billion per annum. Taking the lower death figure of 44,000, this meant that adverse events were the eighth most common cause of death in the United States, ahead of breast cancer and AIDS. Since then, quality has been high on the American health policy agenda. A British government report also looked at the financial costs of adverse events, suggesting that the approximately 850,000 extended hospital admissions that result probably cost the NHS an additional 2 billion pounds per annum. In addition, the NHS was paying around 400 million pounds a year in compensation to victims of clinical negligence (Department of Health 2000a). Following the above, another driver of quality has been a concern to lower the associated costs. As noted in Chapters 1 and 2, a core concern of policy makers across the developed world has been with curtailing ever-increasing health care costs.

While studies reveal the extent of adverse events and medical error, some specific cases of quality problems have also contributed to concerns. In Britain, a public inquiry into substandard performances of heart surgeons at the Bristol Royal Infirmary, which had resulted in multiple avoidable child patient deaths, produced a series of recommendations that have since underpinned NHS policy. As the inquiry report suggested, patients (or their parents) should be involved in clinical decision-making and kept informed, communication with patients should be improved, consent for all procedures should be gained, and health professionals should be open and honest when adverse events happen (Bristol Royal Infirmary Inquiry 2001). Indeed, since 2000, ideas such as making care 'patient centred', of incorporating patient feedback into the 'star rating' system of hospital performance indicators, and of developing incentives to improve service performance have been central to NHS policy (Coulter 2002).

The above cases illustrate the extent of quality and safety concerns in hospital settings. The case of Harold Shipman, a British general practitioner, showed that patients are also at risk in primary care settings. Shipman is suspected to have murdered up to 250 of his patients over a 30 year period but, in 2000, was found guilty of only 15 of these. The Shipman case resulted in calls for greater accountability and monitoring of medical professionals, for ongoing training, and for public disclosure of adverse events when they occur (Horton 2001). The case also highlighted the fact that the regulatory system had failed to provide sufficient oversight of practitioners, or to protect patients from substandard or criminal practitioners. Britain's Chief Medical Officer went as far as to suggest that the General Medical Council, which is responsible for regulating professional standards in that country, took a haphazard approach to disciplinary matters while being 'secretive, tolerant of sub-standard practice and dominated by the professional interest, rather than that of the patient' (Donaldson 2006). Perhaps not surprisingly, there have been widespread calls for reform of the General Medical Council, including from the inquiry into the Shipman episode (Shipman Inquiry 2004). The Shipman case highlighted the lack of attention to ensuring quality within primary care, but it has also had implications for professional organization and clinical governance as discussed in Chapter 5.

Another driver of quality concerns has been studies that revealed the extent of variation in health care. Again, North American researchers have led the way here. The 'Dartmouth Atlas of Health Care' illustrated the extent to which the distribution and utilization of health care differs between regions of the United States. For example, the 1998 Atlas reported that some areas in the country had supplies of physicians and hospital beds well above average, and others well below (Center for Evaluative Clinical Sciences 1998). Similarly, there were widespread variations in the rates of medical interventions for common conditions. Subsequent studies pointed out that variations in intervention rates bore no relationship to the prevalence of illness. It was the opinions of health professionals that determined intervention rates. In other words, different practitioners had different preferences for treatment (Wennberg 1999). These differing preferences and opinions mean that patients with identical conditions can receive quite different diagnoses, treatment advice and prescribed drugs dependent wholly on which physician they happen to encounter.

The identified variations tie in with the concepts of 'overuse, underuse and misuse' of health care which, as noted, the US Institute of Medicine suggested a quality service should seek to reduce. The basic idea here is that variations mean that all three of these occur in health care delivery. Antiobiotic prescribing is an example of overuse, with many countries now making a concerted effort to reduce this. Underuse is where health professionals fail to provide adequate or needed service levels. For example, McGlynn and colleagues found that North American patients they studied received, on average, only 54.9 per cent of clinically indicated care that they required (McGlynn et al. 2003). Of course, this means that many patients will fail to have their health problems identified or managed, which potentially poses higher subsequent costs on the health system. Misuse refers to when services may be provided inappropriately, such as the wrong medicines being prescribed, or services being provided by people who simply are not skilled enough to do so.

A final factor driving quality has been a growing demand from the general public for service scutiny and improvement stemming from cases such as the Bristol Inquiry. The advent of the Internet and related availability of information have also furthered public know-ledge of health services and increased expectations, as discussed in Chapter 4. Coupled with this, governments have worked to formalize and publicize the standards that people should expect from health care providers. An example is the New Zealand Code of Patient Rights which outlines the standards expected of publicly funded health services. This was created following an inquiry into a high profile medical misadventure case in the late 1980s (Cartwright 1988). The Office of the Health and Disability Commissioner is the guardian of the standards laid down in the code and is empowered to investigate public complaints about infringements (Paterson 2002).

THE SOURCES OF QUALITY AND SAFETY PROBLEMS

A considerable amount of research has been undertaken into the different types of quality problems and why they occur. Again, most of this work revolves around hospital care. The main types of errors are listed in Box 3.1. In many cases, where an individual patient has suffered an adverse event, it would appear easy to simply blame the practitioner who is found to be responsible for this. In this respect, the practitioner would be viewed in isolation from the system within which they work and it therefore comes down to ensuring that the prospects for future errors by that practitioner are minimized.

However, when looking at the error types in Box 3.1, many are clearly the result of processes that involve multiple procedures, prac-titioners and parts of a health system. In keeping with this, studies have shown that the sources of error are multifaceted and complex and that most adverse events are actually the result of faulty care systems and processes that lead people to inadvertently make mistakes (Institute of Medicine 2000; Leonard et al. 2004). Even where an individual makes a mistake, the reason is often poor

---

Box 3.1: Types of Error

Diagnostic
Error of delay in diagnosis
Failure to employ indicated tests
Use of outmoded tests or therapy
Failure to act on results of monitoring or testing

Treatment
Error in the performance of an operation, procedure or test
Error in administering a treatment
Error in the dose or method of using a drug
Avoidable delay in treatment or in responding to an abnormal test
Inappropriate (not indicated) care

Preventive
Failure to provide prophylactic treatment
Inadequate monitoring or follow-up of treatment

Other
Communication failure
Equipment failure
Other system failure

Source: Leape et al. 1993.

---

communication, inattention, carelessness or forgetfulness, the root causes of which may be tiredness, overwork and a lack of resources to support optimal performances and teamwork. This means that it is difficult to apportion blame to individuals. The implication, as discussed later in this chapter, is that health care systems require upgrading in order to support improvements in quality and safety.

In addition, accidents and errors often occur in a cascading manner. It may not be any one event that causes a patient death, but a series of circumstances that are not quite right. The British government's adverse events report described a typical such case (Department of Health 2000a: 25–6). A child scheduled for chemo-therapy was accidently allowed to eat before anaesthetic and then admitted to a general ward due to a lack of beds in the specialist pediatric oncology ward. This meant that there were no specialist nurses in attendance. The child's medical records were then mislaid. When it was discovered that the child had eaten, the operation to administer the chemotherapy was cancelled and rescheduled for the next day. However, the surgeon originally in charge of the procedure was to be on leave and there was no proper handover. The next day, the senior registrar then in charge of the procedure was busy elsewhere in the hospital doing ward rounds when called by the anaesthetist to administer the chemotherapy. The senior registrar therefore asked the anaesthetist to perform what was considered to be a straightfoward procedure. Two drugs to be administered, one of which was particularly potent, were not dispatched in accordance with hospital policy. Both of the drugs, which had been delivered together instead of separately, were injected into the child's spine resulting in death. Thus, the case involved several types of errors at mutiple levels of service delivery including communication failures and treatment errors. It also illustrates how the organization of and demands on a health professional's time can contribute to error.

Of course, the sources of error are frequently more simple. Patients are often supplied with incorrect drugs or dosages for reasons such as a dispensing pharmacist being unable to read the messy handwriting of a prescribing doctor.

APPROACHES TO IMPROVING QUALITY

As noted above, in practical terms there are multiple possible approaches to quality improvement due to the fact that quality issues span entire health systems. In conceptual terms, there are two extreme positions that underpin the approaches that might be developed.

First, and sometimes considered to be aligned with neoliberalism, is the 'shame and blame' approach (Liang 2002). This is the idea that practitioners and organizations who are guilty of delivering poor quality services should be publicly revealed. Those found to be responsible for an adverse event or patient death should be named; so should hospitals that deliver poor health outcomes, such as higher post-operative infection and death rates. On the one hand, this approach will inform the public about where they are more likely to receive safe and good quality care and, in theory, it will also drive service providers to improve their quality in comparison with that of others. However, shaming and blaming also carries with it an incentive for practitioners to hide information and deny involvement in adverse events for fear of repercussions. It may even lead to further harm as a result, particularly if a patient has to pursue action through a court or medical council in order to gain an admission of error or even an apology (Wu 1999; Lamb et al. 2003). Revealing information on comparative performances also fails to account for the complexity of medical care. A provider may have a higher post-operative readmission or death rate simply because they have the best surgeons working for them who admit the most complex cases that other providers are loathe to accept. Thus, what would appear at face value to be the worst quality provider may actually be the best.

Second, and closer to social democratic principles, is the idea of 'continuous quality improvement' or CQI. This approach has origins in Total Quality Management as applied to Japanese business in the post-war period (Deming 1986; McLaughlin and Kaluzny 2005). The philosophy behind CQI is that service processes and the activities of people need to be carefully planned to ensure high quality and consistency in service delivery, but also that opportunities for deviation from standards and conditions that contribute to error are eradicated. A core component of a CQI programme is placing a high emphasis on valuing staff, including providing support for practitioners to reflect on processes and to provide feedback that management can use to improve systems and working environments. Management, of course, must be committed to supporting CQI and implementing staff suggestions for quality improvement. Very importantly, CQI hinges on the idea of learning from mistakes, rather than searching for scapegoats. The incentive is therefore to report mistakes routinely and openly, and to not be afraid of doing so. This is so that the contributing factors can be closely studied and understood and systems and processes accordingly adjusted.

Underpinning both the shame and blame and CQI approaches is an emphasis on data collection and the study of work processes so that the activities of practitioners and organizations can be measured and compared with one another and over time. A key challenge with this is the development of performance indicators (Kelley et al. 2006). These need to be carefully designed to ensure that relevant data is captured. There also needs to be care that a focus on data collection does not lead to 'goal displacement' and 'gaming' (Carter et al. 1995). This occurs when a provider organization or practitioners become overly oriented toward producing good results in areas that data are collected for, to the detriment of other activities that are not subject to data gathering, or where they actively cheat the performance management system (Bird et al. 2005). As noted above, a hospital may not want to admit complex cases for fear that complications could undermine perceived performances. Similarly, services may be over-provided to reduce the possibility of complications or complaints.

Clinical guidelines also play an important role in quality improvement for the fact that guidelines have the potential to reduce variations in clinical practice and also to 'close the gap' between how medical practitioners practice and how scientific evidence suggests they ought to be practising (Woolf et al. 1999). A clinical guideline is a dossier of evidence-based information about best practice for the diagnosis and treatment of a specific condition. Hence, the idea that guidelines promote the practice of 'evidence-based medicine'. Naturally, there may be literally dozens of clinical guidelines in existence in any country, depending upon which conditions guidelines have been developed for.

Guidelines development and implementation is occurring in most developed countries today and various methods are used for this. Most common is the consensus method where a group of experts, such as clinicians and researchers, work over a period of time drawing together evidence around best practice. Such evidence includes systematic reviews and the results of randomized trials of interventions or medications. Upon agreement, a guideline will be drawn up. The consensus method has been noteworthy for the considerable resources and time that it takes to produce a guideline. For example, Britain's National Institute for Health and Clinical Excellence 'takes at least 18 months and convenes as many as 15 meetings of the guideline development groups to produce guidance that may need to be reviewed every couple of years' (Raine et al. 2005: 632).

While offering considerable promise for quality improvement, the clinical guidelines movement faces several challenges. These include that available evidence around best practice is often conflicting and incomplete. Guidelines, once developed, may not always provide the best protocols for the treatment of all patients as certain individuals may be better suited to alternative treatment plans. In some cases, guidelines may be used to limit or ration health care, a particular concern in the context of US managed care systems and others seeking to reduce health spending. As such, guideline application could even undermine quality. Finally, clinicians may feel that their professional autonomy – their freedom to do what they think is right

– is being infringed upon by requirements to use guidelines (Woolf et al. 1999). In this regard, guidelines may be viewed as a neoliberal tool designed to increase managerial control.

Of course, researchers and policy makers have suggested a range of practical measures for quality improvement that draw upon different elements of the shame and blame and CQI approaches. The United States Institute of Medicine is a strong advocate, in the context of that country, for a 'system wide' approach that entails a complete redesign of the health system (Institute of Medicine 2001). This, they argue, ought to be at four levels starting with the patient. The first, therefore, would see the system re-oriented with a genuine commitment to being patient-centred by linking it into patient experiences and issues of social justice. The second level would involve changes in the 'microsystems' of care, the teams of health professionals who deliver patient services. These ought to be evidence and knowledge-based, patient-centred and customized to meet patient needs, and built around principles of cooperation. Moreover, key priorities should be patient safety and transparency. The third level was focused on the organizations that house the microsystems. These need to be capable of supporting high quality, safe care by ensuring that best practices become standard practices. The fourth and last level at which change was required was in the external environment including the regulation, funding, professional education, and public policies affecting the health system. In the United States, for instance, the constant threat of medical malpractice litigation poses a barrier to transparency and disclosure among the practitioners who work in microsystems (Wu 1999; Institute of Medicine 2001; Berwick 2002).

Patient-centredness is a theme in other quality improvement studies which suggest that patients should be integrally involved in health system design for the fact that they are able to draw upon their experiences in the process (Bate and Robert 2006). Supporting this is research which shows that patients can identify errors in treatment that are not routinely captured in medical records and so can provide useful information about how to improve quality (Weingart et al. 2005). Research also demonstrates that audit and feedback – the process of informing health professionals about their performance – can improve professional practice (Jamtvedt et al. 2006). There is evidence that shows that a concerted effort to develop a collaborative quality culture among a team of professionals (a microsystem) will reduce the incidence of adverse events (Jain et al. 2006). Finally, there is research that supports the idea of providing financial incentives for health professionals (in essence, a neoliberal construct) to improve the quality of services they deliver (Epstein 2006).

A focus on improving rates of intervention, so that health systems are focused on ensuring that populations receive levels of care that are clinically required, is a strong theme among researchers and policy makers (McGlynn et al. 2003). Comparative studies and projects sponsored by organizations such as the OECD, WHO and the United States Agency for Healthcare Research and Quality are designed to collect a range of population-based data and to systematize clinical practice. The aim is to improve both the process of care (how patients are assessed, diagnosed and treated) and health outcomes by reducing levels of disease and error in the service areas covered. The diseases in question tend to be those that most affect population health such as cancers, vaccines, heart disease, surgical waiting times and respiratory disease (Hussey et al. 2004; Arah et al. 2006; Kelley et al. 2006).

GOVERNMENTS AND QUALITY IMPROVEMENT

Governments around the world have taken differing approaches to improving quality within their health systems. This section outlines developments in Britain, New Zealand and the United States.

Britain

The approach to quality improvement in the British NHS has evolved over time in response to the requirement to adjust the policy framework, as knowledge about its performance has become available when applied in practice, and also as political leadership has changed. The centrally-driven NHS approach includes several developments that are working in tandem and apply to different components of the health system. Being a 'national' health system, the NHS approach has the potential to improve service quality for the entire population.

The first component of the strategy is a focus on developing 'clinical governance' which can be traced back to around 1997 when the New Labour government commenced the process of 'modernizing' the NHS. Clinical governance is discussed in more detail in Chapter 5. Essentially, it has involved clinicians performing a governance role in all NHS organizations with a focus on continuously improving service quality and safeguarding high standards of care through promoting and ensuring clinical excellence (Department of

Health 1998). Accordingly, clinical governance has seen a rejuvenation of professional responsibility for promoting and exacting good service quality. It has also involved increased demands for professional accountability.

The second strand is aimed at service safety and has origins in two reports produced in the early 2000s (Department of Health 2000a; 2001a). In many ways, this is in response to the Bristol Inquiry and related information about adverse events. Thus, in 2001, the National Patient Safety Agency (NPSA) for England and Wales was established. Previously, there were multiple systems for patient safety data collection and so the NPSA was charged with developing a centralized national system which is now connected to over 600 organizations across the NHS. The NPSA system allows for largely anonymous reporting of incidents so as to reduce fear of blame and related hiding of adverse events. Policy makers have also recognized the importance of linking incident reporting to the development of a 'safety culture'. In this respect, a programme to train 'patient safety managers' has been implemented which provides local managers with considerable scope to decide which critical events should be studied for their root causes so that these can be learned from. Challenges include working out how to build a national database of 'root cause analyses' that can be used for professional education (Williams and Osborn 2006).

The third strand within the NHS is a focus on performance improvement. This is partly to do with service efficiency improvement but also quality. The first exercise in applying 'star ratings' was undertaken in 2001. This involved hospitals and ambulance services being given an annual rating from zero for the worst performers, to three stars for the best, as measured against a series of targets. Data on a series of indicators were used for the ratings. These included whether hospitals were able to treat 90 per cent of emergency patients within four hours, whether they were able to reduce the maximum wait time for elective hospital admissions, and whether ambulance services were able to respond to 75 per cent of calls within eight minutes.

There were various problems with the star ratings system, particularly with gaming of the targets by providers so that their performances would appear better (Bevan and Hood 2006) but also that the ratings failed to provide a balanced assessment (Mannion et al. 2005). The system also failed to reduce performance variations among providers (Kmietowicz 2003). In response, the government abolished the system of targets and ratings. In its place, it established the Healthcare Commission, responsible to, but independent of, the Department of Health. The Healthcare Commission is charged with overseeing a new framework of national standards that NHS providers are expected to pursue and against which they will be audited, and also to investigate complaints against service providers (Ham 2005; Klein 2007). Propelling this is the idea that the patients' perspectives should be used to inform service assessments and that national standards will apply to all providers, public, private and non-profit, among which NHS patients are increasingly being given a choice (see Chapter 7).

Lastly, as discussed in Chapter 4, it is anticipated that significant quality improvement will result from the implementation of the NHS Connecting for Health programme. This applies to all NHS providers and facilitates electronic ordering of laboratory tests, prescriptions and electronic patient records, each of which has been shown to provide more efficient information exchange and to reduce the incidence of error (Chaudry et al. 2006). As with many such initiatives, Connecting for Health has not been trouble free and questions remain around whether it will deliver improved quality.

New Zealand

New Zealand's health system has similarities to the British NHS in that it is tax funded, access is universal and public hospitals and services are dominant. When it comes to quality improvement strategies, however, there are considerable differences. These differences mean it is likely that some New Zealanders will receive higher quality care than others.

The New Zealand health system has been through a series of recent restructurings, as noted in Chapter 2. Presently, the central government holds responsibility for national goals and targets for the health system, having devolved service planning and purchasing to a series of local District Health Boards. These, in turn, fund Primary Health Organizations that provide government-subsidized primary care. Like Britain, there has long been an emphasis on developing clinical governance albeit largely in primary care settings, and a key concern among general practice representative groups has been on improving service quality and standards (Malcolm et al. 2002). In 2005, the government introduced a set of primary care performance indicators designed to improve service quality (District Health Boards New Zealand 2005). These are aimed at issues such as improving immunization rates, collecting accurate data and screening for certain conditions, and include a pay for performance component where those collecting required data are rewarded. As noted above, New Zealand has a Health and Disability Commissioner with responsibility for investigating complaints against practitioners and for upholding the Code of Patient's Rights. The Health and Disability Commissioner's office has wide-ranging powers to investigate the circumstances surrounding adverse events. These investigations routinely look at aspects of service management and organization that may have contributed to patient harm and, as a result, it is extremely rare that individual practitioners are singled out (Paterson 2002).

In stark contrast with Britain, the New Zealand government has taken something of a 'hands off' approach to hospital quality, leaving it largely up to individual District Health Boards and hospitals to develop their own improvement programmes and data collection systems. There is a national Quality Improvement Committee that reports to the Minister of Health but this has limited scope for influencing government policy or the activities of service providers. This committee is overseeing a series of projects being 'piloted' by individual District Health Boards, so progress across the system will be variable and problems with comparing hospital performances are likely to remain (Merry and Seddon 2006). A series of basic quality data is collected for all hospitals and produced in a quarterly report (e.g. Ministry of Health 2008). While this is intended to drive hospital performances, it is uncommon for this data to be debated in public or used against a poorly performing District Health Board. In 2007 the government introduced a series of performance targets for District Health Boards largely aimed at improving the delivery of services in areas such as chronic disease management and cancer services (Minister of Health 2007). While the targets have implications for quality, they are not specifically designed to improve clinical quality performance or to promote a focus within hospitals and other organizations on building a quality culture.

In keeping with the heavy emphasis on devolution within the health system, as discussed in Chapter 4, New Zealand does not have a coordinated approach to information and communication technology development. As such, individual hospital and primary care provider organizations have the ability to improve quality for their specific patients through the use of information technology, but at the level of the health system there is limited capacity for coordinated action or information sharing.

United States

Health care in the US is notable for the fact that it is not really delivered via a coordinated 'system' such as the British NHS but, conversely, multiple public and private systems that serve different portions of the population. For patients, the varied nature of health care within a highly fragmented system means that quality is extremely variable. The quality of health care for some well-insured North Americans is among the best in the world. For the approximately 47 million residents with no insurance, service continuity and quality is questionable. Moreover, the sheer enormity of the US system means that the road to quality improvement and application of consistent standards could be long. There has been a gradual acceptance of and push for quality improvement, but market arrangements mean that different funders and providers develop their own methods largely in isolation from one another.

The US government has made an attempt to take a leadership role in quality improvement. Its aim is to focus government-funded health insurers and providers on the issue and, in doing so, to influence activities in the dominant private sector. The Agency for Healthcare Research and Quality (AHRQ), funded by government, is charged with the task of facilitating quality improvement, although initiatives are also funded directly by the Federal Department of Health and Human Services. These include the Hospital Quality Alliance which collects data on a series of measures from some 4048 acute care hospitals. This data reveals that better quality hospitals have lower mortality rates across various recorded measures (Jha et al. 2007). AHRQ funds a wide range of research into quality issues, as well as advocating for health system improvement. It is involved in developing a series of performance indicators that enable comparison between the quality of services among providers and the various US states (Kelley et al. 2006). It is also involved in data collection around patient views of health services and quality and, in this regard, is attempting to change the culture of health care. The objective here is for patients to become more informed when receiving medical care both by asking questions and by being engaged by health professionals. Another area of concentration is promoting the deployment of ICT particularly for improving service coordination and reducing error. Finally, AHRQ is working to improve health outcomes for 'priority' populations such as low income and minority groups that research shows have disproportional coverage by poorer quality services (Fiscella et al. 2000; Hasnain-Wynia et al. 2007).

In 2005, the US government passed the Patient Safety and Quality Improvement Act. This is designed to encourage voluntary and confidential reporting of medical errors to new Patient Safety Organizations (PSOs) that will collect data from multiple providers across both the public and private components of the health system. Using collected information, PSOs are intended to work to develop measures to reduce adverse events and will also be linked into a national Network of Patient Safety Databases (United States Congress 2005). For PSOs to be effective, of course, they need to be in place. By 2008, none had been created which could be due to the fact that creation requires organizations that are willing to volunteer for PSO formation.

Reflecting the considerable variation within the US health system, numerous quality improvement initiatives take place within the private sector. These are highly varied and far from coordinated, while research suggests that only a small number of hospitals have a firm focus on quality improvement (Cohen et al. 2008). Initiatives range from efforts to transform the culture of health care to focus on collaboration, patient centredness and safety (Jain et al. 2006), through to providing practice-enhancing materials and performance data aimed at improving individual practitioner service quality (Meehan et al. 2006). Quality improvement is commonly driven from within a single organization but it is not uncommon for a state-level hospital association (membership of which is voluntary) to promote and provide leadership in quality improvement across its members. Several private for profit and not-for-profit organizations have quality at the centre of all their work. Examples include the winners of national awards such as the government-sponsored Baldridge National Quality Award and the American Hospital Association McKesson Quest for Quality Prize. A prominent theme within many private sector health management organizations, such as Kaiser Permanente, is the application of ICT for quality improvement (see Chapter 4).

Philanthropic organizations and think-tanks also play an important role in promoting quality. A prominent example is the Commonwealth Fund. The Commonwealth Fund has commissioned many studies that highlight quality issues both within the US health system and in comparison with other developed countries (Hussey et al. 2004; Davis et al. 2007). The Institute for Healthcare Improvement (www.ihi.org), funded largely by donors and research grants from Federal government agencies and other funding bodies (including the Commonwealth Fund) is probably the most well-known and active promoter of quality improvement in the US. Its work includes organizing national conferences, running workshops, conducting and commissioning research, and acting as a sometime clearing house for information on quality improvement initiatives. Of course, the Joint Commission, created in the 1950s, has long worked to raise health care provider quality standards. The Commission works with over 15,000 health care organizations and programmes in the US that volunteer to be accredited. Joint Commission accreditation means that an organization has met particular standards (see www.jointcommission.org). The threat of the Joint Commission withdrawing accreditation can act as a strong incentive for a hospital to ensure that it meets basic quality standards. The focus on achievement of standards, however, fails to engender a culture of continual improvement.

CONCLUSION

This chapter outlined why quality and safety are central to the new health policy agenda. It noted that, as a fluid concept, how quality is defined and tackled will depend on the perspectives of the different players involved in the policy process. The chapter also discussed how the divergent approaches to quality improvement – shame and blame and CQI – can be viewed as aligned with neoliberal or social democratic thought. The chapter looked at methods for quality improvement and policy developments in three countries.

As to be expected, there is considerable variation in the approaches to quality improvement among the three countries overviewed in the chapter. Britain's creation of institutions intended to drive quality from the centre, combined with an emphasis on clinical governance and financial performance incentives, represents the most concerted approach. It features a mix of both shame and blame and CQI strategies which ought to drive improvement through the mix of competitive behaviours driven by transparency, as well as the focus on developing learning and improvement focused organizations. This contrasts with the New Zealand and US scenarios. With New Zealand's capacity to command the health system from the centre, the lack of a national strategy or agency to lead quality efforts might be described as something of a lost opportunity. Quality improvement remains ad hoc and largely dependent on locally-driven hospital and primary care initiatives. The US situation is similar but perhaps natural given the fragmented nature of organization within its health care system. However, in contrast with New Zealand, there is more of an emphasis on developing national quality data sets able to be used to propel better performances.

The road to quality and safety improvement remains under construction. All three country examples demonstrate that, in one way or another, quality is firmly on the new health policy agenda. Yet the material in this chapter suggests that much more can and should be done in the interests of patient safety. None of the three countries has considered the sorts of health system reorganizations discussed in this chapter that would support improved care processes and patient safety. Moreover, there are no solid examples of individual hospitals or other services that have reoriented for quality and safety. To be fair, reorganization of the nature advocated by the Institute of Medicine and others would be an enormous undertaking, requiring entire health system or organizational reform. Instead, the focus has remained on improvements within existing systems in areas such as performance management, governance and application of information technology. It remains to be seen whether, over time, these approaches will prove adequate.

QUESTIONS FOR FURTHER DISCUSSION

1. Why is quality an important policy issue, but difficult to define?
2. How might poor quality impact on patients and service providers?
3. What are some of the suggested techniques for improving service quality, and practical initiatives that governments are taking?
4. Is the quality improvement agenda, as outlined in this chapter, a tool of neoliberalism or social democracy, or are there other motivating factors?

4

HEALTH CARE INFORMATION AND COMMUNICATIONS TECHNOLOGY

This chapter explores:

- The varied roles for ICT in health systems, and ways ICT is being deployed
- Why policy makers are interested in supporting health care ICT
- The complex nature of ICT projects and requirements for an effective ICT development
- ICT policy developments in different countries

INTRODUCTION

Information is crucial to effective health care delivery, coordination and quality. This means that information and communications technology (ICT), which includes computers, the Internet, telephones and various mobile electronic devices, has a great deal to offer. ICT is widely utilized in clinical work and, increasingly, is seen as a driver of improved health care organization and of new approaches to service delivery. Indeed, there are high hopes – from policy makers and service providers, through to researchers – that ICT will produce considerable service quality and efficiency improvements, as discussed in the previous chapter, and drive health system transformation. ICT is also changing the way in which patients gain access to health information with increasing numbers now resorting to the Internet for this, and using email and other electronic devices to interact with health care providers. While the promises for ICT are considerable, various circumstances associated with health care, the health sector and available technologies complicate ICT development. Furthermore, governments and health care providers face an array of policy and practical issues that need to be worked through in order to advance ICT.

Of course, the application of ICT and what it means for various actors involved in health care delivery can be viewed in different ways. On the one hand is the idea that ICT is a managerial tool and control mechanism. It has considerable scope for monitoring and systematizing clinical activity and behaviour. It also has potential for improving service efficiency and assisting with the flows of information critical to effective systems and development of service provider markets. In this sense, ICT could be conceptualized as a neoliberal construct. On the other side of the equation, ICT is empowering patients, while driving new forms of participatory decision-making and collaborative clinical activity. ICT could, therefore, be viewed as a facilitator of democratization and community building and central to furthering social democratic aims. As this chapter discusses, developed world ICT strategies incorporate both aims.

This chapter looks at the emergence of ICT on the health policy agenda, why it is important to health care and how it promises to change health care delivery. First, it looks at the role of information in health care delivery. The chapter then discusses some of the practical ways that ICT is deployed in health care settings and the impact of this on health professionals and patients. Third, the chapter looks at some of the policy and technical ingredients required for effective ICT development. Fourth, it overviews the aims of 'high-level' government policy strategies, with particular emphasis on the British case but also New Zealand and the US. The conclusion considers two issues. These are the mix of ICT strategies being pursued by governments, and whether this combination might fulfil the expectations laid down for ICT.

HEALTH CARE AND INFORMATION

Health care is information intensive with all parts of a health system reliant on good information and information systems. Health professionals collect information from patients about their background, presenting symptoms, general health status and recommended course of action. This may include information on drugs prescribed and patient referrals for laboratory tests or to other services. Health professionals are required to keep an up-to-date knowledge of trends and developments in medical practice, pharmacy and research. They are also expected to communicate with one another and exchange information about patients and other issues.

Service funders and managers collect information concerning the volume and demographics of patients treated, types of cases presenting, cost and length of time it takes to provide treatments, service providers involved, service financing and reimbursement, community health care needs, and a host of other information required for planning, decision-making and resource allocation. As noted in Chapter 3, data on quality is an increasing source of information collected by and used for managerial purposes.

Researchers and policy makers have an interest in population-based information that gives insights into issues such as patterns of illness, budgetary trends and service utilization. Patients have an interest in information about their conditions and will collate this from a range of sources including health professionals, friends, support groups and the public domain. The way in which information is collected, collated and, where applicable, transferred between each of these parties (professionals, funders, policy makers and patients) impacts on the relationships between them as well as on the organization, quality and efficiency of health care.

Due to its complexity, health care requires a variety of different forms of information management and systems (Smith 2000). Depending on health system structure, there are multiple possibilities for how information may be collected and managed. For example, patient management systems may exist at an individual practice, community or national level. Individual physician practices, hospitals and the public and private sectors may each operate separate systems. Corporate information may be distributed across a number of sub-national agencies, particularly where service purchasing and planning are devolved to statutory government-funded bodies or non-government organizations. Any developed country can be expected to maintain national data sets (collections of data used to analyse major causes of disease and death, and health care costs). The completeness and reliability of such data sets will be affected by the quality of data collected by service purchasers and providers, whether collection follows a standardized format, and whether submission of data to the national level is enforced.

Traditionally in health care, the paper record has been the core mode of information management, and in many developed countries remains dominant in the keeping of individual patient medical histories. Thus, when a patient encounters the health system, the provider involved (say, a hospital) may need to request information directly from the patient that already exists in paper form elsewhere. Due to difficulties of transferring paper records between, in many cases, a number of health care providers, health professionals routinely perform tests and examinations that may already have been carried out. For the patient and clinician, such duplication and lack of easy access to all available information can be frustrating and time consuming. Funders may view this situation as costly and seemingly inefficient. As discussed below, ICT deployment promises to revolutionize the organization and management of information and of health services.

Research shows that the adoption of ICT varies widely across countries. A 2006 survey of primary care physicians from seven OECD countries revealed that a high percentage of respondents in the UK (89 per cent), New Zealand (92 per cent) and the Netherlands (98 per cent) used electronic health records. While ICT uptake was high, there was wide variation in the extent to which physicians were able to use electronic systems to order and receive test results, prescribe medication, and access patient hospital records (Shoen et al. 2006). This is a reflection of the diversity of systems in use, of the different functions emphasized in the developmental process, and the extent to which different parts of the health system collaborate around ICT development. At the lower end, only 23 per cent of Canadian and 28 per cent of US respondents had electronic record systems. The differing status of development across these countries could at least partly be explained by reference to expenditure on health ICT. As Anderson et al. found, the US was spending $0.42 per capita on ICT compared with the UK investment of $192.79 per capita (Anderson et al. 2006). Of course, there are often widespread within-country variations in ICT application across different parts of the health care system, as various US-specific studies have found (Miller and Sim 2004; Jha et al. 2006; Blumenthal and Glaser 2007; DesRoches et al. 2008).

TRANSFORMING HEALTH CARE: ICT IN PRACTICE

As reflected in various government strategies, ICT can be used in a variety of ways in health care with wide-ranging implications for clinical practice, patient-professional relationships, the future shape of health systems, and for policy makers. This section looks at practical ICT applications and discusses the requirements for their fulfilment.

Electronic health records

At the core of health care ICT is the electronic health record (EHR; also often referred to as an electronic patient record). EHRs promise to revolutionize patient record keeping which, as noted, has traditionally been paper based. Essentially, an EHR is a computerized electronic version of a patient's medical history. The computer basis of the record provides for several possibilities that are often cited by policy makers, clinicians and researchers as reasons for their development and implementation.

The first of these is that the format for the patient record can be standardized. This means that standard EHR software will be used. A hospital may therefore have a single, centralized electronic record system, requiring that information be structured and recorded in a specific format, as may a primary care physician group practice. This contrasts somewhat with paper record systems where different hospital departments may each have maintained their own records and in contrasting formats. Similarly, primary care physician practices may each have had quite different record systems and structures for recording information. Standardization, of course, means that variations in the recording of patient information will be reduced, leading, as studies have shown, to improved data quality (Chaudry et al. 2006). However, it also means that there needs to be agreement on the standards for data collection and recording, on the format and look of the EHR, and on which information should be recorded. Also important is that software is user friendly, reliable and available at the point of service. Obviously, in the EHR software development process, the input of those involved in providing front-line care, especially health professionals, is crucial (Berg 2004). Some may see EHRs as a managerial system designed to control their activities.

Second, email and the Internet mean that EHRs are inherently portable, with the potential to be accessed by anyone with a networked computer. No longer do hospital departments need to wait for paper records from referring primary care providers or other hospital departments, or deal with incomplete information. If EHRs are 'universal' in that all providers in a health system use standard software and have protocols for accessing records, then access will conceivably be instant and on demand. This means a wealth of patient information is potentially available at all points within the system, reducing the need for routine questioning of patients in encounters with new providers about their histories, medications prescribed, laboratory tests ordered and so forth. Portability, however, is surrounded by a variety of conundrums. These include questions about who owns the record system. Will each organization within a health system maintain its own records and allow other providers to access this when necessary, or will there be a centralized system? There are also questions around who should have legitimate access to patient records and whether parts of a record, such as sensitive information on sexual or mental health problems, should be kept private in, for example, a routine encounter for treatment of a common cold at an after-hours emergency centre. Systems also need to be secure so that patients and professionals can have confidence in them.

Third, the portability and potential centralization of EHRs, that, as described above, could form the hub of a patient information system, opens the way for linking into other systems designed to improve health outcomes. In practice, this may involve health providers receiving additional information for particular patients when they open their record during a consultation. For example, a physician seeing a patient of a certain age, body size or ethnicity, potentially at risk of disease, may receive an automatic email reminder to order laboratory tests or screening services, or to offer an immunization or other health check. In this way, an EHR supported health system may improve the focus on population health services and preventive medicine. Of course, an EHR system may also provide automatic reminders to patients about the need for a regular checkup or similar, as mentioned below in a discussion of 'telehealth'.

Fourth, as alluded to above, portability opens the way for patients having access to their own records. A possible advantage of this is that it may empower patients to pay closer attention to their health and health care. It may also provide an element of EHR 'governance' in that patients could have control over which information in their record is routinely accessible. Some EHR systems, such as that in the British NHS, provide a 'my space' component (see Box 4.1, p. 78) that allows patients to insert information into a personalized record. This might be useful where patients want to collect information in one place about their personal health and characteristics. Health professionals may also find this sort of information useful for the fact that personalized records may contain information about how patients react to certain treatments and drugs, or other issues that may be relevant to health care. There is growing usage in various parts of the US of such 'personal health records' (Tang et al. 2006; Pagliari et al. 2007). In some cases these are linked into

EHR servers that will scan personal records looking for entries on particular subjects. In turn, the central server may automatically provide information for the personal health record owner about how they might deal with a condition that they have written about in their record. Where necessary, the central server may also alert health professionals. Again, such developments offer considerable scope for health promotion and preventive medicine, but might also be viewed as intrusive and designed for surveillance and behaviour control.

Fifth, and very importantly, is the assumption that EHRs will lead to considerable cost savings. Studies suggest this will primarily occur through the reduction in expensive medical errors. As noted in Chapter 3, errors result from issues such as failure to correctly read a handwritten prescription, meaning patients receive the wrong medicines or doses. Errors also occur through inadequate communications systems, which EHRs have the potential to counter. But cost savings are also predicted through the greater efficiency that EHRs provide. Research has concluded that North America could save around USD 81 billion annually with extensive EHR implementation (Hillestad et al. 2005).

Sixth, EHRs, along with other ICT developments such as systems that allow for shared financial arrangements, are believed to provide the infrastructural foundation for health service integration. Chapter 1 discussed integration, which paper-based records and information systems have worked against, as high on the agenda for health system organization. The flow of real-time standardized information that EHRs promise offers renewed hope for integration as clinicians and other health providers will inherently collaborate in the building and utilization of patient records. EHRs have also been used to integrate private sector service providers with the public sector. A Singaporean scheme, for example, has seen public hospitals providing EHR software free of charge to private community-based general practitioners. Those participating in the scheme are able to admit patients into public hospitals (patients otherwise would have to be admitted by a hospital-based physician), refer them for specialist consultations, monitor their progress, and receive instant discharge summaries (Gauld 2008a).

Health service support systems

ICT is behind a series of advances that support improved medical practice and service delivery. Every year the volume of medical and health knowledge increases exponentially as evidenced in the number of peer-reviewed publications in medical journals. The Internet facilitates direct online access to such information via medical databases and information services that provide information about best clinical and prescribing practices and new advances. While many medical databases and journals are accessible by subscription only, health provider organizations are increasingly covering such costs to ensure access to the best and most up to date knowledge. This stated, a study showed that the free Google search engine was potentially more useful than traditional sources for medical practitioners seeking diagnostic support (Tang and Ng 2006). Many governments and health organizations also provide their own medical knowledge updates to clinical staff along with electronic guidelines on how to treat specific conditions.

ICT is also driving improvements in information transfer and accuracy. E-prescribing, as noted, is a fundamental of the NHS Connecting for Health initiative and is a central aim for ICT developments in many other health systems (Schade et al. 2006). With e-prescribing, GPs can automatically dispatch electronic prescriptions straight from their desktop computers to a patient's chosen pharmacist. Again, the possibility of misreading and error is reduced. Physicians may also receive automated information at the time of prescribing that will inform them of new knowledge, possible reactions, alternative drugs and so forth. This may increase efficacy and patient safety. The same principles also apply to e-laboratory services, where physicians are able to refer patients for laboratory tests electronically and receive electronic results.

E-prescribing might be seen as one component of what is often called 'telehealth'. This is the application of ICT, particularly portable devices such as mobile phones and hand-held computers but also desktop computers and videoconferencing, to provide services from and to remote locations (Norris 2002). Telehealth services are particularly beneficial to rural communities where specialists can see and talk with patients over video, often with the assistance of a generalist local doctor who may help to describe a condition, and receive their x-ray or other results over the Internet. Telehealth also provides for home-based services. For instance, patients can receive reminders, perhaps by text, to check their own blood pressure and perform other simple tests, and then return these electonically. But telehealth, specifically portable devices, offers other applications such as providing text reminders to patients' mobile phones about their pending appointments. The use of text messaging to mobile phones has also been shown to provide a useful post-discharge support channel (Bauer et al. 2003).

Significant improvements to service delivery are possible with the application of barcoding technology in hospitals where it is well known that patients have multiple encounters with health professionals and associated staff. With barcoding the potential for error is reduced. Tracking technology can provide instant information on patient whereabouts, staff can be sure they are dealing with the correct patient, and data automatically accessible on reading a barcode will provide information on the patient's history and medications (Wright and Katz 2005).

Empowering patients and improving professional-patient communications

ICT has led to new forms of patient empowerment via the revolution in access to information. The main source of this is the Internet which is providing an ever-proliferating volume of health information, the range of which is all-encompassing. From home, a condition-specific search may lead to medical school or physician-provided websites that provide up to date clinical information, open-access academic journals that do not require a subscription, the websites of patient groups, and then various web discussion forums such as chat rooms and interactive websites where people share information about their conditions and experiences. An example of the last is DIPEx.org, a British website, funded largely by donations but run by academics and health professionals. It features video clips of patients' personal experiences with particular conditions such as cancers, mental illness and chronic disease (Herxheimer et al. 2000).

As discussed in Chapter 5, the information revolution, along with changing societal views, has reduced the traditional imbalance between doctors and patients. Patients may often be in a position where they have more advanced or detailed information than their health professional might provide, including a host of perspectives from other sufferers of their condition from around the globe that may range from how to live with a condition through to how best to treat it and likely reactions to drugs. Research shows that patients are increasingly resorting to the Internet prior to consulting health professionals, and taking Internet information with them when they seek medical help (Murray et al. 2003; Dickerson et al. 2004; Valimaki et al. 2007). For such people, the web may fill a need for information and support that simply cannot be provided for in a

10 or 20 minute doctor consultation. Combined with the sheer incapacity for even the most diligent health professional to stay abreast of new trends and drugs, this has led researchers to suggest that doctors may, in future, be information 'brokers' who help patients to understand Internet information and to make decisions about their conditions and treatment (Anderson et al. 2003). It also means that health professionals will need to pay increasing attention to web-based information sources and even help to educate patients around how best to use the Internet. This may be especially so given concerns about the reliability of Internet information sources and the wide range of search results that lay people produce (Eysenbach and Kohler 2002; Eysenbach et al. 2002). For some health professionals, the web may prove to be convenient in that they are able to refer patients to particular websites for further information and support. In fact, it may offer the means for health professionals to manage both swift consultations, yet offer patients comprehensive and high-quality information.

Of course, along with use of the Internet, there is a growing trend of patients directly emailing health professionals. This, too, has empowering potential, but also some practical value, particularly where a patient has a simple request such as a repeat prescription. Studies have shown that some patients prefer email for specific problems as it gives them time to think about how to frame questions, to consider responses and to ask questions that they might feel less comfortable broaching in an in-person consultation (Houston et al. 2004). North American research conducted within the Kaiser Permanente health system, which promotes the use of email between doctors and patients, found that those who emailed had a decreased incidence of outpatient visits (Zhou et al. 2007). Email is also being increasingly used for routine procedures such as booking doctor appointments via web-based systems that show availability of different appointment times. Challenges remain around how health professionals might be remunerated for email consultations (Gottleib 2004).

Further empowering patients, but also spurring health service improvement, is the availability of quality data. Some health systems, such as Britain's and many parts of the United States, are increasingly moving toward placing data on medical errors and health outcomes on the web. The intention is to collect and make such information publicly available in the attempt to drive patient knowledge and choice between different service providers.

Management and planning systems

ICT has long been essential to the management and planning of health services. Indeed, there is evidence to suggest that, in mainstream public services, managerial purposes have been the primary motivation for ICT application (Chadwick and May 2003). In health, ICT is used for financial management, managerial communications, and for management information systems. Information systems are particularly important for decision-making and policy makers around the world are increasingly highlighting the need for robust data collection which ICT provides for. In practice, this means requiring that front line health providers (who may see this as a managerial demand) and their employing organizations collect and input specific data about patients and services provided. In so doing, national population datasets can be built.

Such data may be used to calculate costs and understand services provided and also assess overall service quality and appropriateness. Planners and decision makers, for instance, may be able to access how many people have suffered from particular conditions, or required certain services, as well as how many have not accessed services such as immunization or cancer screening programmes. They may also be able to extract information on patient body size, nutrition, drugs prescribed, medical errors, and a host of other issues that may be useful for planning. Key to this, of course, is the design and completeness of data collection and the compliance of front line service providers as data collectors. Busy health professionals may view demands to collect routine data as a distraction and burden and it may be that certain incentives (financial or other) will be required for the additional work (Casilino et al. 2003; Anderson et al. 2006).

Management uses also include the analysis of routine data in areas such as hospital throughput and patient outcomes. Comparative data may provide insights into the relative efficiency of services and extent to which these are improving patient health. Again, management may use such data by making it publicly available in order to drive improved performances. An example of this is New Zealand's elective services league tables that are published quarterly (www.electiveservices.govt.nz). These show how many patients are awaiting elective treatments in each public hospital, how many patients fail to be treated within the government's targeted timeframes, and how many services use nationally-consistent methods for prioritizing patients.

INGREDIENTS FOR EFFECTIVE ICT DEPLOYMENT

It is not uncommon for health care ICT projects to run into trouble. This is partly as ICT projects are typically highly complex and involve a diverse range of technologies, people and agencies, but also because of a series of basic factors that are pivotal to success (Dalcher and Genus 2003; Royal Academy of Engineering and British Computer Society 2004; Gauld 2007). These factors are particularly important in the context of governments attempting to implement national system-wide health information strategies. They are also important to organizations embarking upon ICT projects, as discussed below.

There is evidence to suggest that the extent to which existing hardware and software systems have been coordinated and are 'interoperable' will have a bearing on how practicable the development of future coordinated ICT systems will be (Anderson et al. 2006). Interoperability is a term that describes whether computers can communicate perfectly with one another and is an aim of all health information system planners interested in service coordination and collaboration and issues such as EHRs. A lack of intereoperability creates difficulties for sharing and transferring information and can even endanger patient safety if data is corrupted during transfer.

To achieve interoperability means attention must be paid to coordination of 'system architecture'. Numerous combinations of computer hardware and software exist, supplied by a range of competing companies. Naturally, without central oversight and coordination, health agencies will make what they deem to be ICT purchases appropriate for their purposes, or they will develop their own 'in-house' systems. Often, systems in place have been purchased or developed for specific purposes such as patient record keeping. Where various systems are in existence, there is a high likelihood that there will also be multiple different forms of data collection, classification and coding which confound the quest for interoperability. With key lessons for health ICT policy makers, and coinciding with social democratic sentiments, studies have shown that coordinated system architecture standards result in improved interoperability and reduced ICT expenditure (Kuperman et al. 2000). Conversely, government failure to coordinate ICT developments has been shown to counter interoperability and create a set of circumstances that are especially difficult to rectify as has been the case in New Zealand (Gauld 2004). This is because of the embedded nature of computer and software systems that require costly and labour intensive work to alter.

An effective network that allows information sharing between providers and organizations requires a high level of data security to protect against hackers and build user and patient confidence in the system. Security in health care can be difficult to achieve, especially in busy hospital settings. Clinical staff often want immediate access to information and simply leave systems logged on. Thus, while systems may be hacker resistant, data may be openly accessible. As such, secure systems may also require simple log-on processes and enforcement of system-wide security policy.

As with security, the protection of personal information and privacy is critical. Research suggests that the public have concerns about electronic data privacy and EHRs (Goldman and Hudson 2000; McDonagh 2002). Policies need to be developed around collection of, access to and protection of personal information and the public needs to be involved in this process. Once developed, such policies need to be widely disseminated and strictly observed to bolster public trust in ICT systems and information sharing (Smith 2000; Berg 2004).

Also required is coordination of data standards including the type of data collected, the form this is collected in and the way in which electronic information is sent. There are numerous possible combinations of diseases and complaints. When information is shared, it is critical that common definitions are used. The WHO has promoted the use of ICD-10 (International Classification of Disease Version 10), to ensure a common international language. For electronic data exchange, HL7 (Health Level Version 7) has become the agreed international standard. Obtaining complete compliance with such standards is a critical challenge for full interoperability (Hovenga and Lloyd 2002). Yet even with international standards and widespread support for these, variants exist. In recognition, there are both international and national working groups aiming at ICD-10 and HL7 standardization (see, for instance, www.hl7.org; www. who.int/classifications/icd/en).

Usually, it will not be enough to achieve all of the above. In fact, an ICT project or system probably will not be successful unless it is aligned with the needs of end-users, and system performance will be contingent on their behaviour. User resistance has been found to be key factor in ICT project failures (Gauld and Goldfinch 2006; Gauld 2007). The lesson here is that health professionals need to fully accept and want to use a new computer system, device or software package. This is where involving them in project development is critical. In parallel with this is the requirement for project leadership which, in health, needs to be provided by people with a strong understanding of the technical, organizational and clinical implications of ICT. Of course, the messages that the benefits of ICT policies and related changes are likely to deliver are additionally important. In this respect, politicians may have a key role in clearly explaining policies and how they relate to practical service delivery. Finally, an ICT project may require an element of 'organizational reengineering' (Berg 2004). EHRs and other health ICTs are likely to demand new ways of working that cross professional and organizational boundaries and this means that traditional barriers to information sharing and collaboration need to be traversed. This, in turn, may demand organizational reconfiguration and even health system restructuring.

GOVERNMENT HEALTH INFORMATION STRATEGIES

Since the late 1990s, several of the developed world's governments, seeking to harness the potential of ICT, have issued ambitious and wide-ranging health information strategies (see for example NHS Executive 1998; Advisory Council on Health Infostructure 1999; National Health Information Management Advisory Council 1999; WAVE Advisory Board 2001). Such strategies largely focus on applying ICT to issues of service integration and quality improvement, but they also aim for improved management systems, efficiency and accountability. This section highlights the typical arguments and objectives that various government strategies contain, focusing on the examples of the British NHS, New Zealand and the US.

Health information strategies have often coincided with government promotion of 'e-government' more generally (e-government is the application of ICT to improve and revamp public services delivery; Heeks 2006), and have been developed in response to various health sector issues. The first of these issues is the fact that ICT deployment has been rapidly increasing in health care settings. Second, because governments have wanted to ensure that ICT developments are coordinated. As discussed above, ICT is quite unlike other health policy areas in that developments which are not coordinated are difficult to rectify. A third reason is that governments view ICT as having the capacity to transform and generally 'modernize' the health system.

The British example

In 1998, with *Information for Health*, the British New Labour government was among the first to issue a health information strategy. *Information for Health* set out the government's vision for ICT and forged the path that present policy directions have built upon. The document, which was an 'information strategy for the modern NHS', had an overriding objective of harnessing information to ensure that:

> patients receive the best possible care. The strategy will enable NHS professionals to have the information they need both to provide that care and to play their part in improving the public's health. The strategy also aims to ensure that patients, carers and the public have the information necessary to make decisions about their own treatment and care, and to influence the shape of health services generally
>
> (NHS Executive 1998: 9)

In pursuit of these objectives, *Information for Health* detailed the government's commitment to developing electronic health records for every patient. Once developed, the idea was that all NHS health professionals would be able to access patient records online at any time, along with information about best clinical practice. *Information for Health* also pledged that patients would receive 'geniunely seamless care' as GPs, hospitals and other community providers would share information across the NHS 'information highway'. Patients would also have swift access to information and services, enabling self-care, through Internet service delivery and the development of telemedicine and other services such as call centres. Finally, there would be more effective use of NHS resources through health planners and managers having improved access to information. This would occur as a result of improved data collection, access and transfer, as well as the availability of information routinely inputted into computers by NHS health professionals and agencies. Financial management would also be enhanced by using 'e-commerce' systems to pay for goods and services such as consumables and salaries.

The British government has remained committed to these ideas with some natural additions as its NHS ICT and modernization programmes have evolved. For instance, in 2001 the government highlighted the requirement for various information collection, security and privacy standards, and reiterated the need for electronic health records (Department of Health 2001b). It also stated that ICT would drive an initiative where patients needing surgery or a specialist consultation would be able use the Internet to 'choose' a hospital of preference and then 'book' an operation time. As discussed in Chapter 7, this has been pivotal to the idea, rooted in neoliberalism, of giving patients choice between competing providers, both public and private. Allied with this was the idea that the Internet would facilitate access to information about service performance that would be published online. Such policies, of course, were designed to make services more 'patient centred', to encourage patient involvement in decision-making, and also to drive provider performances. In this sense, they might be seen as satisfying both neoliberal and social democratic ideals.

In 2002, the 'National Programme for IT' in the NHS was launched with a goal of developing an integrated ICT infrastructure for all NHS organizations by 2010. The objectives of this programme include development of a national ICT system including connectivity between all GPs and hospitals, electronic prescribing – where prescriptions are emailed directly to dispensing pharmacists – and electronic referrals for laboratory and other tests. The NHS programme remains one of the world's largest ever ICT projects and, as discussed below, has not been without problems. Initial costs were predicted to be around GBP6–7 billion. Part-way through the project, in 2007, the NHS estimated that final costs would be around GBP12 billion, but others have suggested it could rise significantly above this (National Audit Office 2006; NHS Connecting for Health 2007) as cost overruns with such large projects are endemic (see the discussions in Standish Group 2001; Dalcher and Genus 2003; Royal Academy of Engineering and British Computer Society 2004). Four separate private ICT contractors are involved in developing the National Programme for IT. Oversight of the programme is presently the responsibility of an agency known as 'NHS Connecting for Health'. Some of the existing and planned components are listed in Box 4.1.

Other country strategies

As noted, Britain is not alone, with the governments of Canada, the United States, Australia, New Zealand and others also issuing health information strategies. Like Britain, core aims include developing electronic health records, accessible from anywhere by anyone with a legitimate right to do so (including patients) and able to be added to as necessary, and the development of national information system

---

Box 4.1: Examples of NHS ICT initiatives

NHS Direct Online (www.nhsdirect.nhs.uk)
This website portal provides comprehensive information on healthy living, illnesses, conditions and treatments. The website has an interactive healthcare guide and regular feature spots providing detail and further information on specific conditions and health issues. Examples include a focus on depression developed in conjunction with the Centre for Evidence Based Mental Health at Oxford University. This presented the first ever guide to depression, interactive tools for recognizing symptoms, evidence-based treatment summaries and audio/video material. A 'find your local health service' feature on the website is designed to help people locate service outside of normal opening hours. The website also features a 'self help' section which allows people to search by symptoms, and provides suggestions on where to go for further assistance. Also included in NHS Direct is a health encyclopedia and a section that provides answers to numerous common health care questions.

nhs.uk (www.nhs.uk)
Like NHS Direct, nhs.uk provides a range of information about the organization of NHS services and in many ways is the gateway to the range of NHS websites. It allows for users to search for health information, and for local providers, provider information and service priorities. Nhs.uk provides links to sites that feature provider performance data, and also allows for patients to choose among providers and book appointments online.

National Library for Health (www.library.nhs.uk)
This is a comprehensive electronic library for use by clinical staff. It provides regular 'evidence' updates, and links to key evidence and other databases such as the Cochrane Collaboration Library, various clinical guidelines and associated services, and medical databases and journals.

Healthspace (www.healthspace.nhs.uk)
This secure website allows patients to develop their own personalized health record including information such as height, weight and blood pressure. It is freely available for use by any NHS patient over the age of 16.

---

standards. Also strongly emphasized is that ICT will improve quality, efficiency and patient-centredness, as well as integrate the disparate parts of the health system and facilitate universal access to considerably more information. In many cases, governments or health care purchasers are linking financial performance incentives to ICT development and provider usage for the fact that quality and efficiency improvements can be expected (Rosenthal et al. 2006; Campbell et al. 2007).

New Zealand

While the aims of other governments might be comparable to Britain's, the process of implementation differs. In New Zealand, the government has taken a more passive approach. The centralized planning approach of the NHS programme does not align with the New Zealand government's preference for devolved planning and policy implementation. A historic lack of central oversight of New Zealand ICT developments, especially in the 1990s when health care regions and providers were expected to compete with one another, means an array of different ICT and information infrastructures centred around the 21 separate District Health Boards and 80 Primary Health Organizations is now in place (WAVE Advisory Board 2001; Gauld 2004). These have been established by a mix of private ICT providers and 'in house' developers. Thus, while utilization of ICT in New Zealand health care settings is high, as noted earlier in this chapter, and many primary care physicians have highly sophisticated electronic systems that incorporate guidelines, decision-making and other quality improvement tools, the capacity for interoperability and for developing portable EHRs remains low.

At present, there remains no policy or plan to develop standard EHRs. For the most part, this is due to the complexity and cost of integrating or replacing the existing disparate ICT systems. However, New Zealand also has yet to work through the debate around whether EHRs can be shared among providers. This means that a primary care physician who happens to consult with their own patient outside of hours, but in a separately-owned after-hours facility, will only be able to access information on the patient collected during prior visits to the after-hours facility. They cannot access their own records on the patient, or any other patient's usual records. The government, for its part, has issued a strategy that contains a series of long-terms goals although it has recognized that it is not in a position, due to the embeddeness of existing systems, to create a national ICT infrastructure. Instead, it has taken the stance that it will help coordinate attempts by service planners and providers to develop collaborative and interoperable systems and provide support for developing national ICT standards (Health Information Strategy Steering Committee 2005). In short, while there is significant potential for ICT to improve health care quality at the level of the individual provider and hospital, owing to the penetration of ICT across the health sector, there is restricted capacity for implementation of coordinated ICT-driven quality improvement initiatives. The ability for ICT to drive integration is similarly limited.

United States

The US federal government has refrained from issuing a full-blown strategy for health ICT, but has attempted to propel the development of EHRs, the uptake of which, as noted earlier in this chapter, is low by international standards. In 2004, President George W. Bush issued a statement that EHRs would be central to quality improvement, to improved patient experiences with services and to the future organization of health care. Bush outlined a ten year plan for EHR implementation designed to reduce health care costs while also improving quality. The plan included developing national health information standards, investing in demonstration projects to identify best practices that might be adopted on a national basis, use of government agencies to lead in the adoption of EHRs, and requirements that agencies purchase interoperable ICT systems (Bush 2004). It is likely that President Barack Obama, inaugurated in 2009, will advance the promotion of ICT which was a centrepiece of his pre-election health policy plan.

EHR uptake remains patchy and slow (DesRoches et al. 2008). However, publicly-funded agencies such as the Veterans Health Administration have long been leaders in the field having, in 1999, launched the development of a national EHR system across the 21 service networks that deliver care for its patients (Oliver 2008). ICT is viewed as having been pivotal to the transformation of the Veterans Health Administration into an integrated and quality focused health system. In 2007, the Promoting Health Care Information Technology Act was introduced to Congress. If passed, this will establish a National Coordinator of Health Information Technology, will authorize the Health Secretary to make funds available for the purchase of interoperable ICT systems, and develop a Health Information Technology Resource Centre. Like Britain, the legislation also aims to facilitate public-private partnerships for ICT development. Looking ahead, one of the key challenges for the US will be promoting the conditions that are conducive to ICT adoption. Research suggests that this could require not only financial assistance and incentives, but also that larger physician organizations are more likely to use electronic record systems (Rittenhouse et al. 2008). ICT implementation could well create a demand for physician group consolidation.

CONCLUSION

This chapter detailed developments in health care ICT. It looked at why ICT is important to the health policy agenda, including envisaged transformations at multiple levels of health systems. The ICT developments described in this chapter might be viewed as responses to practical issues and as simple applications of newly available technology aimed to improve administrative and service delivery systems. They may also be viewed as having the potential to satisfy neoliberal demands for managerial control, facilitating choice and performance monitoring, as well as social democratic aims for building collaborative working arrangements, bringing services and the public closer together, and improving health care quality. The chapter discussed the complexities of ICT projects and the ambitious ICT strategies of developed world governments, as illustrated by the example of Britain.

The three country cases overviewed in the chapter illustrate a variety of approaches to ICT. Britain's system-wide project holds considerable promise and, in many ways, adheres to what is known about best practice for such undertakings. The government has taken a leadership role, it has a clear set of aims and has maintained central control over the project and the standards for ICT. On the downside, the sheer enormity of the project means that there have been implementation problems, which could carry high financial costs and have implications for its future performance.

The New Zealand and US examples differ considerably from that of Britain. New Zealand shows how ICT developments across a health care system can take on a life of their own if the government or a specific organization does not proactively coordinate these. As a consequence, the New Zealand case is unfortunate. While ICT has been widely adopted, interoperability is low, limiting the possibilities for health system transformation. There is restricted scope for ICT facilitating provider collaboration or public engagement. Being something of a laggard in ICT adoption, especially with regard to EHRs, the US faces an enormous challenge in that it needs to dramatically expand ICT utilization across its health sector. This will require a considerable financial investment, as the British government has committed to, but it also provides an opportunity to ensure coordinated developments with greater potential for getting the foundations in place for interoperability, clinical data collection, quality improvement and patient involvement. A key issue for the US, with its low capacity for central government leadership in health care matters, will be whether it is able to develop and implement a British-style coordinated strategy, or follows the New Zealand path where government has assumed a largely hands-off approach which facilitates incremental yet parallel developments. Of course, as noted in this chapter, a criterion for successful ICT implementation is involvement of health care professionals throughout the process. As the next chapter discusses, the rise of clinical governance has been assisting with this.

QUESTIONS FOR FURTHER DISCUSSION

1. What sorts of ICT applications might be the most useful for improving health care?
2. Which issues do policy makers need to consider when planning for a successful ICT development?
3. Is the application of ICT likely to satisfy a neoliberal, managerialist agenda or facilitate better collaboration and coordination and, therefore, improved patient experiences?
4. Which of Britain, New Zealand and the US has a higher likelihood of implementing a robust ICT system?

5

GOVERNANCE, PROFESSIONALISM AND PUBLIC PARTICIPATION

This chapter explores:

- Concepts of governance and clinical governance
- The changing nature of health care professionalism, and the influences behind the changes
- How patients and the public are involved in health care planning and decision-making processes in different countries

INTRODUCTION

Governance has become a focal point in health policy debates in the post-neoliberal era. This has been partly in the effort to rectify difficulties with managerialist structures but also in response to quality and safety failures and the desire to promote clinician involvement in improving health system performance and in issues such as information technology development and utilization.

In essence, 'governance' describes arrangements for governing the organization and management of health services and health professionals. The term 'clinical governance' has often been applied to health care governance arrangements specifically aimed at improving clinical services and service quality. Clinical governance structures may involve health professionals as well as the public. Indeed, in keeping with social democratic ideals, public participation or public involvement in health care decision-making and planning is often viewed as central to good clinical governance.

Clinical governance policies and arrangements have had wide-ranging impact on the shape of health systems, including on the nature of 'professionalism' which itself has evolved in response to a changing professional practice and service delivery environment. In some cases, clinical governance has rejuvenated professional practice and organization, especially where doctors have been involved in forging new strategic directions for service delivery and improvement. In other cases there is evidence of a new divide where institutions designed by the state or by managers for the governance and monitoring of professional practice and service delivery have been poorly received by front-line health professionals. This has been so because of two developmental directions. One, harking from the neoliberal stable, has seen increasing accountability, monitoring and control of professional behaviour. The other direction, with social democratic underpinnings, involves increasing the patient voice and formalizing this through governance structures, in turn posing challenges to professional power.

This chapter discusses the rise of health care governance, of demands for responsiveness to the public and patients, and of patient involvement in health service governance. The chapter looks predominantly at the British case as it has been at the forefront of changes in these areas, but also at New Zealand and the US. First, the chapter overviews the concept of governance. Second, the chapter looks at the emergence of clinical governance. Third, the changing nature of professionalism is discussed. Fourth, the chapter considers the trend of patient involvement in health care decision-making. The conclusion discusses whether changes in governance, professionalism and participation will improve health systems and health care.

WHAT IS GOVERNANCE?

Governance has become a policy focal point in many countries. The term is widely used across the gamut of public services, yet its definition and application remain broad. In general, governance describes structures for governing services. As such, governance structures may involve a governing board and management team, usually with input from the public, front line professional staff and others as required. The term 'governance' is also often used to describe one of the aims for structures for governing the activities and performance of health professionals. Governance activities are usually carried out with the support of a full-time secretariat that may include a chief executive and other support staff who, in turn, may oversee an organization such as a hospital. Governance structures will, therefore, include a 'top' level group of people (a governing board or committee) with specific expertise or skills that allow for them to provide guidance and to scrutinize the work of the full-time secretariat. This can lead to tensions, especially where the governing board fails to agree with the perspectives or advice of full-time officials. Of course, a governing board for a public service may be under the tight control of central government (the 'shareholder') and so the board, in turn, will place pressure on officials to perform in certain ways.

Governing board activities will generally include setting strategic directions for an organization, developing or approving policies, and monitoring operational performances. A governing board may be structured in different ways. A 'corporate' structure in the neoliberal tradition would usually feature a solely appointed membership of people experienced in governing private businesses. It would operate largely out of the public view and be focused on financial management and organizational efficiency. Consultation with the public or with health professionals and other front-line service delivery staff around decisions would be minimal, and there would be considerable use of formal contracts and financial incentives to exact improved performances from staff.

In contrast, a 'democratic' or community-oriented governance structure may be composed of elected and appointed members with the aim of facilitating community input into the decision-making process. Appointed members, for instance, may be there for their experience in community work. Board meetings may be open to the public in the spirit of transparency, and there may be widespread consultation with implicated or interested parties in all governance activities. There may also be extensive use of contracts, performance incentives and other mechanisms to increase the accountability of front-line staff. Governance, of course, is also central to the organization of professional groups such as doctors. The structures will reflect particular circumstances and aims, but most professional bodies are governed by members elected from within the profession. Such bodies may also include appointed members or lay people to provide broader representation and input.

It is sometimes suggested that public service governance as described above is about 'governing without government' (Rhodes 1997; Peters and Pierre 1998). What is meant by this is that there is an emerging form of government in which central government provides broad strategic policy directions, while local or group-based 'governing' bodies work through the detail of developing specific policies, creating accountability structures, and monitoring peformances. In this sense, 'governance' represents a recognition that policy is not strictly a top-down affair, controlled and administered by central government. It is also a practical manifestation of devolved decision-making, especially where governance bodies are ultimately responsible to central government for performances within their jurisdiction or for the way public money is spent. The resulting structures are a recipe for complexity as multiple governing bodies may be individually responsible for services in their respective areas. They may be required to compete for improved performance yet collaborate with one another around national service delivery goals and services that intersect regions.

THE RISE OF CLINICAL AND HEALTH CARE GOVERNANCE

Governance is not a recent phenomena. Hospitals and health services in developed countries have long featured governing boards of varying sorts. Health professionals have traditionally been involved in these as well as in the administration of hospitals and health services. More recent is the increasing prominence of the concept in health policy discussions. Indeed, governance has been on the agenda in the British NHS since at least 1997 (Scally and Donaldson 1998). It has also been central to policy in places such as New Zealand, Hong Kong, many European Union countries, and Pakistan (Shiwani 2006). Essentially, governance, particularly the idea of 'clinical governance', has been a response to a range of issues. First, to preceding organizational arrangements founded on neoliberal ideas. As noted in Chapter 1, these involved creating market-oriented arrangements for health care delivery that included corporate governance structures as described above. The emergence of social democracy has brought with it the community-oriented concept of governance in explicit recognition of a desire to broaden the scope of involvement in health care planning and decision-making. However, as noted above, the emphasis on accountability and monitoring has remained with, perhaps, renewed vigour. In this way, governance, in contemporary terms, has both democratizing and performance improvement and accountability aims.

Second, the focus on governance has been advanced by the quality improvement and patient safety agenda (see Chapter 3). Thus, underlying governance concerns have been the various studies showing high rates of medical error, and the high profile cases of misadventure that have gone undetected. The errors and lack of systems to monitor professional practice are a consequence, it is often suggested, of poor service and professional governance especially around the extent to which health professionals are competent to practice and have adequate systems for self-regulation. The underlying assumption, therefore, is that improvements to clinical governance would result in better quality and safer health care. Of course, central to clinical improvement are health professionals themselves who have been at the heart of the new clinical governance movement.

Clinical governance has significant potential to impact on professional practice and organization, as well as patient outcomes. Certainly, the clinical governance rhetoric in Britain, discussed below, is that professionals are critical to a team-building approach focused on raising standards and leading service improvement. Other countries have seen a similarly strong movement towards involving medical practitioners and other health professionals in service governance.

The British example

An illustration of the above, indicative of changes in process in other health systems, can be found in developments in Britain. As Chapter 3 discussed, a series of inquiries into health system failures produced recommendations that there should be a more systematic approach to quality that empowered patients and involved clinicians in improvement efforts (see, for example, Gray and Donaldson 1996; Nicholls et al. 2000; Bristol Royal Infirmary Inquiry 2001; Shipman Inquiry 2004).

Such recommendations were represented in the idea of 'clinical governance' which was a core component of the New Labour government's NHS 'modernization' agenda. Clinical governance was described by the government as 'a framework through which NHS organisations are accountable for continually improving the quality of their services and safeguarding high standards of care by creating an environment in which excellence in clinical care will flourish' (Department of Health 1998: 33). It has been suggested, and given the emphasis on 'accountability', that clinical governance was to be a management-led system 'designed to set and monitor clinical standards' which was an activity the NHS had not previously engaged in (Salter 2007). Furthermore, clinical governance was to involve the government in working to clarify which treatments work best, again in the effort to reduce variation and eradicate outmoded practices. In practice, the new framework meant that the tradition of professional self-regulation would remain in place, but that the NHS would work to develop systems to ensure self-regulatory bodies were open to public scrutiny, responsive to changing patient needs and clinical practices, and publicly accountable for the setting and monitoring of professional standards (Department of Health 1998). In sum, both neoliberal and social democratic sentiments were enveloped in the new directions.

Among the difficulties with implementing clinical governance was the very fact that it was a broad concept, and there was limited understanding of how best it ought to be put into practice. Moreover, the concept was being applied from the top-down across the entire NHS. Accordingly, clinical governance involved a national managerial and regulatory framework, but also extended to professional self-regulation. As Salter notes 'clinical governance was at various times taken to include medical audit, clinical audit, critical incident reporting, adverse event reporting, risk management, annual appraisal, and quality assurance – in other words, anything which could be understood to maintain and improve clinical standards' (Salter 2007: 265).

The government's response was to create a series of new regulatory and monitoring arrangements, with differing functions but no national coordination. This said, a new Clinical Governance Support Team based within the central government Modernization Agency was responsible for providing aid to NHS organizations in their governance development processes. New institutions included the National Institute for Health and Clinical Excellence (NICE). This was designed to appraise new drugs and medical devices, provide guidance on treatments and procedures, develop clinical guidelines and, very importantly, develop clinical audit tools to aid health professionals in their clinical governance activities (Rawlins 1999). To provide a framework for monitoring and evaluating the work of health authorities, a set of National Service Frameworks were developed. These prescribed evidence-based best practice for certain chronic diseases and patient groups. The Healthcare Commission, which initially used a system of 'star' ratings, was created to carry out inspections of local hospital clinical governance performance and to report back to NHS planning and funding organizations. In practical terms, for NHS hospitals and health care providers, a good star rating for clinical governance meant an effective and collaborative system of leadership had been created, including a vision and set of values that had been communicated to all staff. It meant specific plans for quality assurance and improvement had been developed, such as ensuring that staff were receiving appropriate education and training and capable of delivering high quality services. It also meant collecting data on clinical performance and using this to highlight variations, as well as redesigning work processes for improved service delivery and involving the public in this (Halligan and Donaldson 2001).

Various studies provide insights into the process and impact of implementing Britain's new clinical governance arrangements. Freeman and Walshe surveyed governing board members and directorate level managers in 100 NHS trusts about their views on the achievement of the various clinical governance expectations outlined above. Their findings indicated that clinical governance structures appeared to be well established. However, there had been better progress with quality assurance which was reflective of the performance management culture being driven by central government institutions. This was at the detriment of quality improvement, meaning that the rhetoric of quality improvement coming from central agencies was not being reflected in practical developments. There was also no evidence that organizations subject to review by the Healthcare Commission were performing any better than those that had not been (Freeman and Walshe 2004). A related study found that there was inconsistency in the processes of reviewing clinical governance applied to different NHS trusts, and in the resulting action plans developed by trusts in agreement with the Healthcare Commission. Again, the focus of governance reviews was more on management processes than on direct patient care and outcomes (Benson et al. 2006).

Other studies have looked at the implementation of the clinical governance policy at the service delivery level. Hogan et al. found that medical specialists they interviewed had mixed attitudes. Some felt there was an absence of a common approach to quality improvement, of a focus on improving inter-professional relationships, or of clinical engagement by management. Others, working in a hospital where there were clear structures and processes for supporting staff, where management was open to suggestion, and where communications across all staff groups was seen to be effective, had more positive attitudes toward the clinical governance programme. All interviewees felt that availability of time to focus on improving governance was a significant barrier (Hogan et al. 2007). Resourcing for clinical governance, which is aimed at influencing the way people work in health organizations, was the focus of a study that found management was generally not providing adequate support for human resourcing needs required to deliver on the policy (Som 2007).

Clinical governance experiences in New Zealand and the US

Britain's difficulty with putting clinical governance concepts into action is not unique, although it could be a function of the managerially-driven top-down nature of the implementation process. If so, it may be that there has been insufficient attention to ensuring professional involvement in shaping the change process. Elsewhere, there are examples where health professionals have led the way from the 'bottom-up' with clinical governance development.

In New Zealand through the 1990s – interestingly a period of neoliberal government – over 80 per cent of the mostly sole-charge general practitioners formed into networked organizations. This was largely to facilitate the process of negotiating service contracts with purchasing bodies. These new Independent Practitioner Associations, as they became known, quickly recognized the benefits of organization. However, toward the latter part of the 1990s, as the government gradually began to embrace social democratic health policy aims, there was support for the new associations developing in new directions. As with British primary care trusts, many of the associations negotiated bulk funding for services delivered and were able to keep any surplus funds for investment in new patient services and supporting infrastructure. Association governance was by elected general practitioner and practice nurse members. Very important was an equal focus on clinical and financial accountability. Research suggests that this professional-led model of clinical governance was rewarding for health professionals, that it reinvigorated general practice, and produced many positives for patients by way of expanded scope of primary care services. Key lessons from the New Zealand experience appeared to be that clinical governance works best with minimal bureaucratic control but appropriate accountability structures, and that personal financial incentives were less important than ability for clinicians to use savings to improve and expand the range of health care and preventive services (Malcolm and Mays 1999). Subsequent developments have seen the government attempting to subsume the Independent Practitioner Associations under new Primary Health Organizations. This has met with mixed success, with some of the clinical governance gains of the 1990s reversed (Gauld and Mays 2006; Gauld 2008b).

In the US, there is naturally considerable diversity in terms of governance structures, with hospitals being a mix of state or local government-funded 'public' institutions, private non-profit or for-profit organizations, all of which feature governing boards. These boards vary widely in structure, they are predominantly appointed or elected from within the ranks of the organization, and their focus is primarily on income generation and profitability. There are, however, models of management-professional 'partnerships' which are comparable with aspects of governance developments in Britain and New Zealand. A well established example can be found in California's Kaiser Permanente which, over a period of 50 years, has built 'an organisational culture that transcends the traditional conflicts between "medicine" and "management" ' (Crosson 2003: 654). This culture has been founded on principles of joint leadership and acknowledgment of mutual dependency, careful alignment of managerial and physician objectives so that both are focused on a common set of values, and a commitment to providing management training for medical professionals so that they can work as 'truly effective partners in the management of their practices' (Crosson 2003: 654).

In US primary care, the ownership and governance landscape is diverse and not conducive to the centrally-driven promotion of clinical governance that has been possible in Britain. Primary care organizations can include specialists as well as general 'family medicine' practitioners. In organizational terms, a proportion of primary care organizations have been labelled 'integrated medical groups' which tend to be larger and have clinical governance structures. The US also features 'individual practice associations' which are loose networks of otherwise independent and often sole practitioners. Research shows that the integrated medical groups tend to deliver higher quality care (Mehrotra et al. 2006), but that probably only one third of primary care practices have clinical governance structures and team-based approaches to care in place (Rittenhouse et al. 2008). This poses a substantial challenge for the US not only in terms of promoting clinical governance and team work, but also as 47 per cent of all private primary care practitioners work in small practices with only one or two physicians. Furthermore, the numbers of practitioners in larger integrated practices has not increased over time (Bodenheimer 2008).

It could be concluded that clinical governance has played a role in rejuvenating medical practice and professionalism in the wake of neoliberalism. It could also be asserted that the concept has been one of a number of challenges, especially for the medical profession, that is shifting the power balance between government, health professionals and patients, and that is contributing to an evolving agenda for professional regulation, organization and behaviour. The next section considers the changing nature of professionalism.

GOVERNANCE AND EVOLVING PROFESSIONALISM

The medical profession, as an elite group, has a particular place in health policy. It has traditionally been the most powerful provider group with often unrivalled access to policy makers. There are a range of reasons for this including a monopoly on medical knowledge and protection of this that a professional association provides, the crucial role of medical practitioners within health systems and corresponding threat of strike action if they do not get their way, and public sanction – the deference that lay people have given to doctors as all-important and not to be questioned (Jones 2003). The power in policy debates of a national medical association, that licenses and represents all medical practitioners, has traditionally been such that politicians tread carefully – often consulting closely with the profession – when crafting policy.

This traditional professional power, however, has been gradually eroded as society has changed. Over time, the public have become more vocal about what they want from doctors, partly driven by the culture of consumerism. There has also been a growing perception that professional standards have been in decline (as noted above and in Chapter 3). The Internet has revolutionized the traditional knowledge imbalance that favoured medical professionals. People are now able to access an exhaustive range of medical information on the Internet and communicate with others about diagnoses and the sorts of treatments available.

Neoliberal policies, of course, were an attack on established interests and promoted the idea that individuals (patients) should have choice and primacy, while managerialism sought to subsume professionals under new management control structures. A range of developments in clinical practice have impacted on professional autonomy. These include the rise of evidence-based medicine and idea that all practitioners should follow evidence-based guidelines for best practice (see Chapter 3). In this way, variations will be reduced, quality and safety increased, and clinical practices systematized. Formal processes for prioritizing patients by scoring them against predetermined clinical criteria serve similar purposes (Siciliani and Hurst

2005). The emergence of new government regulatory bodies, as described in the previous section, poses particular challenges to professional power and organization with the imposition of new levels of monitoring. Finally, the boundaries of various professional groups have become blurred. Some countries have allowed for nurses to prescribe certain medications. Some medical specialties have encouraged others with lesser qualifications to conduct routine procedures in their fields (Nancarrow and Borthwick 2005). In response to such challenges, and of course the emergence of clinical governance, the nature of professionalism has evolved.

Evolving professionalism in practice

Britain has been leading the way with redesigning the governance of professional standards. In other countries, similar changes are underway, but these have not been as strongly advocated for, nor the effort as concerted. In Britain, the threat of government intervention led the General Medical Council (GMC), the organization that oversees the range of professional colleges, to seek redesign of the governance of professional standards. Indeed, it has been argued that the government focus on patient safety is posing a significant challenge to medical regulation. This is due to the fact that quality concerns have given policy makers and managers a legitimate reason for collecting data on professional performances, and for driving higher standards and regulatory change. This, in turn, has prompted the medical profession to take ownership of the safety and quality agenda (Waring 2007). The GMC began this process in 1995 with the launch of its *Good Medical Practice* guide, intended to lay down new standards for clinical training and practice (General Medical Council 1995). It also increased the number of lay people on the GMC and developed a new approach to assessing incompetent doctors with the input of lay people.

By the late 1990s, the GMC was advocating for a 'new professionalism', suggesting that professional self-regulation – where specialty colleges regulate their own members, set their own standards and (often closed-shop) processes for hearing cases of misadventure – was no longer good enough. What was needed were new regulatory parameters that would focus the profession on leading and upholding clinical standards, on putting patients first and involving them in all decision-making processes, and on development of collegial 'team' approaches to peer review and quality improvement. The GMC saw as its core task to shift the professional culture from one of self-protection and solidarity to a culture of 'professional quality improvement' that 'combines professional, managerial, and patients' perspectives' (Irvine 1999). In this way, the aim was to satisfy neoliberal accountability and performance expectations, and social democratic concerns about patient-centredness.

Debates over the shape of medical professional regulation have been ongoing, particularly around professional revalidation. This would require all doctors to show that they are fit to practise as judged against a series of standards including medical knowledge, clinical skills and capacity to communicate with patients. Resistance by some professionals to the idea of assessment led to initial revalidation proposals being watered down (Irvine 2005). In 2007, a government white paper outlined a process for annual appraisal using a '360 degree' feedback tool that gathers performance information from a range of sources including NHS employers, colleagues and patients, with the onus being on practitioners proving their competence to practise (Shaw et al. 2007). This, it is suggested, is a model of 'partnership regulation' with patient safety at the centre (Bruce 2007).

Britain is not alone in pursuing the idea of a 'new professionalism'. Similar concepts are under implementation within Australian medical colleges responding to a 'growing culture of suspicion whereby professionals are no longer trusted to regulate themselves', with lay appointments and a focus on continuing education (Lawson et al. 2005). In New Zealand there is also said to be a new professionalism emerging 'with clinicians becoming collectively and professionally accountable for both the quality and cost of their decisions, in a new and successful form of clinical autonomy' (Malcolm et al. 2003: 654). Similar trends can be found in Italy and Sweden as well as other European Union countries (Quaye 2007; Lega and Vendramini 2008).

In 2005, in reponse to 'changes in the health care delivery systems in virtually all industralized countries [that] threaten the very nature of and values of medical professionalism', an alliance between the European Federation of Internal Medicine, the American College of Physicians – American Society of Internal Medicine, and the American Board of Internal Medicine produced a physician charter (ABIM Foundation 2002). This called on doctors to renew their sense of professionalism by committing to lifelong learning, being honest with patients, and ensuring that all receive a uniform and adequate standard of care. The charter also urged doctors to eliminate educational, financial, geographic and social barriers to accessing services. The charter was criticized for failing to advocate for genuine collaboration between medical and allied health professionals, such as nurses and public health practitioners, and for failure to suggest partnerships with health care provider institutions (Reiser and Banner 2003). Yet, in the context of managerial demands for improved accountability, the charter was seen by its authors as an affirmation of important traditional medical values.

The wide range of ideas behind new professionalism create significant challenges for the future of medical education and regulation. There are questions around who should be accountable for the competency of doctors: professional associations, employers, or government regulators? Moreover, there is a need for medical professionals to have additional skills in management and in communications, in group (team) work, in understanding how to extend services to more deprived populations, and in techniques for functioning in a 'performance-based' environment. In the light of this, Klass has suggested that judgements of professional competence will increasingly depend on 'situational' evidence that draws together a holistic account of a practitioner's involvement in the process of care. Again, central to this is the perspectives, experiences and outcomes of patients (Klass 2007). All of this, of course, could place further pressure on doctors who are increasingly busy and in short global supply (World Health Organization 2006; OECD 2008b). Professionals disgruntled at additional and new methods of monitoring could simply voice their concerns by shifting countries. As such, governments and regulatory bodies need to proceed cautiously. Experiences and progress with public and patient involvement, a key theme in clinical governance and the new professionalism, are the subject of the next section.

PUBLIC AND PATIENT INVOLVEMENT

Since the late 1990s many developed countries have been promoting the involvement of the public and patients in the planning and delivery of health care services, although ideas of involvement and participation are not new (Rifkin 1981). Public involvement generally refers to the idea of involving members of the public in strategic planning and decision-making about the funding and configuration of services. The term patient involvement is usually applied to measures to involve patients, along with health professionals, in decisions about individual treatment and care (Florin and Dixon 2004). Given the complexity of health care systems and services, there is the potential for public and patient involvement policies to be difficult to implement. This is partly due to the wide variety of possibilities for involvement and extent to which these are controlled by health professionals and managers, with limited geniune scope for change and influence. Yet there are strong arguments for involving people in service development and decisions around individual treatment options.

These include that if people are paying for services, for example through taxes, then they should be involved in shaping them. This perspective aligns with the neoliberal concept that, without such accountability, service providers will place their interests ahead of the public interest. At the service planning level, involvement could be by a genuinely representative sample from the community. In keeping with this is the argument that more democratic decision-making leads to improved public accountability and is an inherent public good. There may be substantial benefits with public involvement around ethical issues so that community values are taken into consideration. Public involvement initiatives may also be seen to benefit the public by ensuring that services are made more responsive and oriented toward improving public health and health care quality. This in turn, it is often suggested, may lead to improved health outcomes. Underlying many public involvement policies is the idea that only the public know what is best for them, and that the views of professionals and managers may fail to represent these (Florin and Dixon 2004). There is also the notion that the trend toward public involvement reflects attempts to counterbalance the 'democratic deficit' in democratic politics that has seen a decline in voter participation in general elections along with reduced trust and faith in political leaders. In a similar manner, public involvement may reflect a shift away from purely neoliberal constructs and service planning arrangements.

The arguments for patient involvement are generally that patient compliance with care instructions will be improved as a result, and that the increasing numbers of patients with chronic disease requires 'self-care' strategies that can be developed in conjunction with patients. Such strategies entail encouraging patients to become more involved in controlling their own health care and behaviour. There is also the argument that patient involvement policies are a response to higher patient expectations (Fudge et al. 2008). As Arnstein's work suggests, there are varying degrees of participation in decision-making (Arnstein 1969). Full and genuine participation often means a transfer of power to the public or patients which may be resisted by managerial and professional staff. In such cases, participation may be tokenistic and unlikely to result in patient-centred partnerships between professionals and patients.

How people should be involved remains an imprecise exercise, with a wide range of suggestions (Wait and Nolte 2006; Chisholm et al. 2007). Key public involvement channels include elected membership of boards, commissions or bodies that provide feedback to service planners or undertake service planning. The idea is that such mechanisms will ensure representation and advocacy on behalf of electors. Public involvement may be facilitated by the creation of specific institutions charged with receiving input from the public, but not necessarily involving elected membership. Where lay people are involved they may be selected on the basis of their experiences (perhaps in community service provision or advocacy) or skills. Of course, elected or appointed organizations may canvass the public to ensure that they have received the full range of opinion and that any advocacy or decisions adequately reflect real-life experiences. Such consultation may be conducted by way of surveys, public meetings, visits to specific groups or communities, or by inviting submissions from the community on specific issues. Public involvement mechanisms also include citizens' juries, where, like a court of law, invited (usually randomly selected) members of the public hear evidence for and against a certain policy and then offer a decision. Such decisions would be unlikely to be binding, but are intended to provide a representative 'citizen' view to inform policy-making.

Patient involvement can take a myriad of shapes and forms (Crawford et al. 2002; Florin and Dixon 2004). Again, patients may be involved in providing feedback on service configuration or performance. Central to this may be service satisfaction surveys or forums where patient representative groups provide advice to service providers about patient experiences to ensure that services are responsive to patient needs and meet expectations. At a less formal level, patient involvement is integral to quality improvement efforts and to effective clinical practice. Professionals need to be sure that they focus on patient needs and include others such as families in the process. They may involve patients in the process of diagnosis, but professionals also need to be sure that advice is considered to be appropriate and that patients feel comfortable about disclosing information that could be crucial to the care process. Similarly, many chronic care patient involvement initiatives will revolve around specific care plans developed in conjunction with the patient.

Various studies have looked at the impact and potential of public and patient involvement initiatives and the requirements if they are to be effective. A systematic review found few studies that explored the actual impact of patient involvement initiatives (Crawford et al. 2002). Around three quarters of studies reviewed were individual service case studies, meaning that it was difficult to draw generalizable lessons from the results. There were no studies that looked into the effects of involvement on health, quality of life or service satisfaction, leading to the conclusion that there was no evidence to suggest that participation improved health outcomes. However, there was evidence that involvement initiatives can lead to changes in service configurations such as making services more accessible or providing better information to patients, and that those participating in involvement initiatives often reported a positive experience (Crawford et al. 2002).

Another study looked at the way in which health services in the British NHS interpret user involvement policies, and which factors influence how these policies are put into practice (Fudge et al. 2008). The findings were that health professionals were largely leading the development and initiation of involvement policies and this potentially limited the extent to which involvement initiatives could influence change. There tended to be more patient involvement in less technical areas and areas where clinicians were less involved in service delivery. The explanation for this was that public and patient involvement concepts were understood in different ways by different people and professional groups, and driven by personal ideologies, needs and different contexts (see also Thompson 2007). In Arnstein's terms, discussed above, this meant public participation in many cases was closer to tokenistic and more likely to involve professionals simply providing information (Arnstein 1969). Significantly, the research found that only small numbers of service users were 'involved' and that personal gains – such as feeling listened to by health professionals, the opportunity to meet other patients with similar conditions, and to learn more about the services available – accrued from this (Fudge et al. 2008). Of course, such a finding suggests that patient involvement could perpetuate inequalities. Comparable findings were produced by a Canadian study which found that there was a 'significant gap' between the intention to involve patients in health planning and their actual involvement. This was due to a lack of clear guidance for how patients should be involved, a dominance of service providers in planning activities, and other priorities that took precedence over patient involvement (Gold et al. 2005).

Other studies imply that involvement initiatives have the potential to clash with 'evidence-based' service delivery (Harrison et al. 2002). In this respect, there are suggestions that involvement policies are unlikely, by themselves, to be an effective way of improving professional accountability and service quality (Baker 2007). Studies also indicate that there is little consistency in the methods used for involvement. Furthermore, that public representatives often have difficulty grappling with who it is they are meant to be representing, meaning that the range of 'views' contributed could potentially be quite restrictive, and that they sometimes find the required commitment to 'being involved' demanding (Florin and Dixon 2004).

In terms of what the public might want from involvement initiatives, research suggests that people like to be listened to and see evidence that their voices have been heard (Anton et al. 2007; Hogg 2007). Some would rather not be 'involved' in decisions about their treatment (sometimes as they are too unwell), preferring to place their trust in professionals (Thompson 2007). One study implied that involvement in decision-making was more appropriate at the planning and service development level than the individual patient level, but that consultation, without responsibility for final decisions, ought to be the aim of such processes (Litva et al. 2002). It may be that coaching could be required for more effective public and patient involvement. Indeed, research shows that tailored coaching can help the way patients interact with health professionals and lead to better individual health care and outcomes (O'Connor et al. 2008).

Several studies report on the findings and experiences of citizen juries and deliberation processes. These show that citizen views on issues such as funding prioritization may well alter as a result of hearing evidence. Studies show that deliberative processes can have significant consequences for health policy, particularly if an 'informed' public, able to learn more about an issue through deliberation, is able to help steer decision-making (Abelson et al. 2003). Having heard the evidence and arguments of government policy advisors and medical experts, one citizen jury came to the conclusion that a policy already in place to screen women aged 40–49 for breast cancer was not appropriate (Paul et al. 2008).

Public and patient involvement in practice

Britain has, again, been at the forefront of pursuing public and patient involvement policies, although recent initiatives are simply the latest in a succession of policy changes. The first efforts commenced in 1974 with the creation of 185 independent Community Health Councils (CHCs) which were local partly elected and partly appointed bodies intended to provide community input into the work of NHS managers. CHCs were established amid much excitement and intended to offer a channel for scrutinizing and improving the NHS. However, their relevance gradually declined particularly during the neoliberal era.

In 2000, the *NHS Plan* proposed abolishing the CHCs but, amid resistance to this, the government simply restructured the mechanisms for involvement. This entailed the creation, in 2003, of a Commission for Patient and Public Involvement, charged with promoting patient and public involvement, and with assisting the administration of a network of some 572 appointed local patient forums linked to NHS trusts. These arrangements lasted only a short time, following concerns about the performance of the Commission for Patient and Public Involvement. In 2006, further restructuring saw the introduction of a new set of 152 appointed Local Involvement Networks (LINks) that had similarities to the earlier CHCs in that they were locality rather than NHS trust based. Unlike CHCs, however, the new LINks have no statutory rights to information or to inspect NHS services and many questions about their role and the extent to which they might contribute to local democracy remain unanswered (Hogg 2007). The succession of reforms has probably undermined the development of involvement mechanisms. Through serving to confuse the public, as reforms routinely do, public confidence in and knowledge of structures has undoubtedly been affected.

A 2008 report by the Local Government Association Health Commission suggested further reforms to enhance local accountability of the NHS. Such reforms, the Commission noted, are desired by central government to ensure that there is local accountability for variations in service performance. They would also serve to shift accountability within the NHS away from central government. If implemented, the Commission's recommendations could eventually see a wide range of commissioning (purchasing) work being subject to scrutiny by local communities and their representatives (Local Government Association Health Commission 2008).

Elsewhere, there have been similarly mixed objectives for and experiences with involvement initiatives. For example, New Zealand's District Health Boards (broadly similar to NHS trusts) are designed to involve the public in health care decision-making and feature a mix of elected and appointed members. Yet the regulatory environment has determined that these boards are under firm central control and accountable firstly to government. The Ministry of Health routinely provides education to board members about their responsibilities for implementing government policy. Because of this, some boards have collectively agreed that members should not speak out about issues without endorsement of the entire board. Voter participation has remained well below 50 per cent, considerably under the 70–80 per cent turnouts for national elections (Gauld 2005b). However, District Health Boards are required to consult with the public in all their work. Their meetings are open to the public, they routinely hold public forums to discuss issues, and invite submissions on policies under consideration. Despite this, there has been a low level of public interest in participating in board work.

Perhaps expectedly in the US, there are no national policies for patient involvement and involvement is not common in the planning and delivery of services. However, a small number of hospitals and medical groups do actively seek to involve patients in their work. Examples include the coopting of patients onto the advisory boards of various services at institutions such as Massachusetts General Hospital. The boards of some hospitals, such as the Children's Hospital of Cincinnati, routinely commence their meetings with patient stories and involve patients in board work. Other hospitals involve patients in board planning retreats, meet regularly with patient groups, and have established a 'patient and family advisory committee'. The US does feature routinely collected national data from the Consumer Assessment of Healthcare Providers and Systems surveys funded by the Agency for Healthcare Research and Quality (see www.cahps.ahrq.gov). This data is presented in combination with clinical performance data (see www.hospitalcompare.hhs.gov). This Hospital Compare data, as it is known, is intended to be used by health insurers and the public to assess hospital performance and, ultimately, to aid decision-making over which providers to patronize. However, it is unclear how insurers and providers use this data to improve patient experiences, and the public and patients are generally not involved in this process.

CONCLUSION

This chapter overviewed policy developments in clinical governance, professionalism and public involvement. These three areas are intertwined for the fact that they have at their centre relationships between government, health care professionals and the public. These relationships are in transition as policies and practical arrangements continue to evolve.

The developments discussed in this chapter may simply be viewed as natural responses to practical issues. These include demands by professionals for involvement in service management, for increased professional accountability in the wake of medical misadventure cases, and for more public voice in service governance and planning in keeping with rising patient expectations and knowledge about services. They might also be seen as responses, in a social democratic context, to preceding neoliberal arrangements, as may be the case in Britain and New Zealand.

The approaches to the issues covered in the chapter differ among the three countries; they are in their infancy, yet broadly similar directions can be found in each. In Britain, concerns for performance improvement motivated the range of new service monitoring and governance bodies, as well as the quest for new professionalism. Britain's changes have also been about bringing professionals back into the decision-making arena and, through patient involvement initiatives, highlighting local accountability. New Zealand's early primary care clinical governance developments were a sector response to central government policy, while regional planning structures have been intended to facilitate public involvement. Notably, the US differs for the fact that developments have lacked government intervention, and patient involvement does not widely feature. However, there is increasing pressure to expand clinical governance, build a more responsive health care system and involve the perspectives of patients in this.

Britain's policies remain a work in progress and it is unclear whether they will produce envisaged improvements. The continual changes in the three policy areas discussed in the chapter could serve to be counterproductive and erode confidence in the NHS among both providers and the public. Professionals, driven by requirements to achieve measureables, and subject to new forms of public and managerial scrutiny, could compete against the 'system' to perform well. On the upside, such assessment processes may improve responsiveness to peer, patient and public concerns. If so, then a new era of quality-focused medicine built around partnerships between providers and patients could emerge. Initiatives such as the European-American physician charter could also help foster such directions.

Of course, drawing policy lessons is a fraught endeavour (Rose 1993). The example of US integrated medical groups demonstrates the positive results that can come from clinically-led clinical governance developments. These groups also illustrate the need to locate examples of good practice and then work to extend these across health systems. Doing so in the US remains a considerable challenge which a British-style government drive could assist with. But whether top-down policy has been beneficial for Britain itself is questionable. Better results there may have come from a central facilitation of clinical leadership and development as in the early New Zealand experience with primary care clinical governance.

QUESTIONS FOR FURTHER DISCUSSION

1. Why is clinical governance an important concept, and what is hoped to be achieved by its development?
2. What are some of the reasons for the emergence of 'new professionalism', and will new professionalism improve health care?
3. What are the benefits and disadvantages of patient involvement policies?
4. Are clinical governance and 'new professionalism' more likely to serve a neoliberal or a social democratic agenda?

6

PUBLIC HEALTH, HEALTH DETERMINANTS AND DISEASE CONTROL

This chapter explores:

• How views about public health and health determinants have evolved over time
• The concept and impact of 'new public health' on the policy agenda
• Prominent public health issues in the new millennium including globalization, health inequalities and chronic disease

INTRODUCTION

Public health is a core part of the health policy jigsaw within the national borders of any country as well as at a global level. Yet public health has long taken second place behind policy and expenditure related to personal health services. This is reflected in the budgetary allocation to public health which, across OECD countries, ranges between 2.5 to 7 per cent of total health expenditure (OECD 2008).

There are various reasons for public health's 'backseat' position. The key one is that personal health services are delivered to patients presenting with directly observable needs such as acute illnesses (for example, a heart attack) and injuries. Such services tend to be associated with hospitals and medical specialities and also include community based general medical practitioners and are largely delivered to individuals who present with a health problem. Most personal health services, therefore, are aimed at diagnosing and rectifying medical conditions. In contrast, public health is focused on populations – neighbourhoods, cities, regions, countries and even the world – and is about developing group or area-based programmes to promote good health and well-being among the individuals involved. Because of this population focus there is also a political underpinning to public health in that its aims and scope, and related interventions, are often determined not by observable need but by the views of governments and politicians and the demands of groups. Such views have evolved over the years, along with the relative prevalence of neoliberal and social democratic ideals, as have the issues deemed to be central to public health and the approaches to health improvement.

Since the 1990s, public health has been moving up the policy agenda of developed world governments. This has been in response to various issues. First, has been a growing recognition that a strong focus on public health ought to reduce pressure on personal health care the demands for which, as noted in Chapter 1, have been growing. Second, views about the scope of public health, and its underpinning philosophy, have progressed to encompass a range of economic and social factors in what is often referred to as the 'new public health'. Many governments pursuing social democratic aims, along with international agencies such as the WHO, have come to acknowledge and promote these ideas in policy-making. Third, a range of new issues facing societies – from the rising incidence of obesity and other non-communicable diseases, through to global warming and new infectious disease outbreaks (e.g. Asian bird flu and SARS) – have brought new challenges which require policy responses.

This chapter overviews developments and issues in public health that are at the centre of the new health policy agenda. Examples are drawn from various countries, including Britain, New Zealand and the US, to illustrate different government responses. The first section looks at the changing understanding and scope of public health and ideas about what it is that determines the health of a population. Second, the chapter discusses issues that are central to the public health agenda today, including globalization and the challenges of inequalities and chronic disease. The conclusion revisits the different ways that countries have responded to the public health agenda and whether these responses are adequate.

THE EVOLUTION OF CONTEMPORARY PUBLIC HEALTH IDEAS AND PRACTICE

Various definitions of public health can be found. As Beaglehole and Bonita note, what these have in common is 'the idea that public health is defined in terms of its aims – to reduce disease and maintain health of the whole population – rather than by a theoretical framework or a specific body of knowledge' (1997: 145). In keeping with this, public health is a wide-ranging field. It includes:

- strategies or programmes to prevent and guard against specific diseases. These may be communicable diseases, such as tuberculosis or SARS, or non-communicable as in the case of heart or respiratory disease and cancer;
- health education and promotion including programmes designed to improve understanding of how to prevent the spread of diseases such as HIV/AIDs, as well as campaigns to improve mental health or nutrition and exercise; and
- government regulation of factors that influence health. Examples include tobacco, drug and alcohol control, the enforcement of seat-belt use in cars, and controls on emissions of air pollutants and noise.

Underpinning the above is a basic understanding of the causes of ill health and how to improve this which is where research, especially epidemiology, plays a crucial role. Of course, ideas around how to deal with many public health issues (for example, improving levels of exercise among a community) may be open to debate and there may be limited research evidence to draw upon when attempting to develop policy initiatives (Nathan et al. 2005). Moreover, there may be a diversity of views about what ought to be considered public health issues. This is a theme that has endured the history of public health (Tesh 1995). There have been tensions between narrow medical perspectives concerned with the 'science' of public health (epidemiological, statistical and laboratory sciences), and the views of advocates for a broad-based 'community development' approach to public health (including influencing socio-economic determinants of health, behaviours, lifestyle and urban environments; Baum 2008). There have been tensions also between neoliberal perspectives on public health (that individuals should take responsibility for this), and social democratic views (that government has a responsibility for citizen welfare).

From the founding of modern epidemiology in the 1850s, when

John Snow established that cholera had been spread via the handle on a water pump in London's Broad Street (Cameron and Jones 1983), medical advancements and personal health services were viewed as responsible for improvements in health. Challenges to this emerged in the work of McKeown (1979). Based on analysis of mortality data, McKeown argued that declining mortality and corresponding increases in life expectancy commenced prior to major medical discoveries of the late nineteenth and early twentieth centuries. Improving health was the result of non-medical factors including better living standards and nutrition. Szreter subsequently challenged McKeown's argument suggesting that people's living conditions would not have improved without the involvement and regulation of the state. Furthermore, that health improvements in Britain and elsewhere occurred in parallel with increasing civic pride and state development. Szreter's work emphasized that the state does have a role in improving public health (Szreter 1988).

The work of McKeown and Szreter was important in the context of parallel developments occurring from the 1970s onward as governments, researchers and others started to embrace the fact that a range of non-medical determinants were crucial to health improvement. Canada's Lalonde Report of 1974 encapsulated such ideas (Lalonde 1974). This proposed that medical and health services were one of four 'fields' that influence health, the others being environment, lifestyle and human biology. The Lalonde Report's impact in Canada was limited but it commenced an international debate around the role of non-medical determinants (Beaglehole and Bonita 1997: 215).

The WHO Alma Ata declaration of 1978 added weight to the debate with its commitment to 'health for all' by the year 2000, again through focusing on non-medical determinants (World Health Organization 1978). The key to achieving this was seen to be primary care development. Other elements of the WHO declaration relevant to public health included a need for member countries to:

- recognize that health status was influenced by and intertwined with social and economic development and encourage a comprehensive approach to improving health;
- develop health promotion and disease prevention strategies and involve all sectors of society and the health system in this;
- aim for equity in health status; and
- encourage participation in the planning and organization of community based primary care.

The foundations for what is commonly called 'new public health' were laid with the 1986 WHO Ottawa Charter for Health Promotion which was motivated in part by recognition that numerous countries had failed to implement the Alma Ata recommendations. The Ottawa Charter was, again, underpinned by beliefs that good health depends on a stable environment, and on good employment, income, food, shelter and social justice (World Health Organization 1986). It was aimed at socio-political issues and provided an often cited five-point framework for health promotion (see Box 6.1).

Box 6.1: The Ottawa Charter's Framework for Health Promotion

- Develop healthy public policy. Such policy would recognize that most policies affecting health fall outside the traditional concerns of the health sector and its agencies. Healthy policies would include free, universal education, legislation to protect the environment and occupational health and safety, progressive taxation, comprehensive welfare, and control on the sale of harmful substances such as alcohol and tobacco. Following this, health would become a concern of all government agencies.
- Create supportive social, economic and physical environments aimed at helping people to reach their full potential as healthy citizens.
- Strengthen community action. This referred to activities that raise the ability of people to change their physical and social environments through collective organization and social action.
- Develop personal skills. These skills would be aimed at helping people to make healthy choices, assuming that behaviour and lifestyle influence health. Such skills would also be extended to community organizations and those involved in lobbying and advocating for improved conditions.
- Reorient health services. Here, the focus of health systems would be moved from personal hospital-based and high technology treatment services to a concentration on community-based and controlled, user-friendly services focused on upstream health improvement (World Health Organization 1986).

The Ottawa Charter was succeeded by a series of publications further elucidating new public health ideas and showing how these differ from traditional public health (e.g. Ashton and Seymour 1988; Peterson and Lupton 1996; see Table 6.1). Since the 1990s, there has been increasing government recognition that the key public health determinants are social, cultural and economic (e.g. National Health Committee 1998). This was reiterated in the 1997 WHO Jakarta Declaration (World Health Organization 1997).

Despite these developments, as noted in Chapter 1, this was also a period in which neoliberalism was in vogue and so in many cases such advice was poorly received. Furthermore, policies in areas such as housing, welfare and the organization of health services often worked in counterposition to new public health philosophy. Examples of this include measures in countries such as New Zealand to reduce availability of subsidized public rental housing (to boost the private rental market and reduce state responsibility), to reduce welfare benefits (so as to provide incentives for beneficiaries to enter the workforce), and to promote competition in the delivery of public

Table 6.1 Traditional and new public health compared

Traditional Public Health	*New Public Health*
Improve physical infrastructure, particularly sanitation, housing and water	Improve infrastructure but also social services and support, communities, behaviours and lifestyles
Medical profession central to public health	Medicine one of many contributors to intersectoral public health action
Expert dominated with some community involvement	Emphasis on community participation and partnership
Epidemiology	Multiple research methods and ways of exploring health improvement
Focus on disease prevention and health as absense of illness	Disease prevention and health promotion focus with health positively defined
Prevention of infectious and contagious disease	Concern with all health threats including environmental and physical such as chronic disease
Improving conditions of the poor	Equity is an explicit policy goal

Source: Adapted from Baum (2002: 36)

health care services (to reduce cost and increase efficiency and patient choice; Boston et al. 1999; O'Brien 2008).

New public health has come to the fore in the new millennium, partly in response to a pendulum swing in politics away from neoliberalism, but also due to increasing evidence showing that action is required around issues such as reducing health and other inequalities, improving housing, promoting comprehensive primary care and changing the way people live. A series of broader issues around the relationship between people and the planet have also driven concern for public health as discussed below.

PUBLIC HEALTH IN THE NEW MILLENNIUM

This section looks at the changing context for public health via a series of issues at the top of national and international policy agendas.

Globalization

Due to the processes of globalization, national and international concerns are becoming progressively intertwined. In-depth discussions of globalization can be found elsewhere (for example Held and McGrew 2000; Kaul et al. 2003). Essentially, the relevance of globalization to public health is in the interconnectedness occurring with increasing international flows of capital, people, goods and services. This is in addition to the rapid transfers of disease that international travel facilitates, as well as the transfer of ideas about public health organization (Beaglehole 2003).

Globalization means an increasing role for international governance and agencies and for agreements between nations about issues affecting both the planet and individual countries. It means a need for countries to act in the global interest, and for global responses to issues likely to impact on domestic health. In this regard, the emergence of new infectious diseases has provided challenges. The 2003 SARS outbreak illustrated how swiftly infectious disease could be transported between countries. As the epidemic unfolded, national governments and the WHO worked to implement surveillance and control systems. Hong Kong and Singapore, for instance, declared states of emergency and resorted to quarantining victims and their contacts (Abraham 2005; Gauld 2005c). It emerged that the 'Westphalian' system for global governance, established in 1648, in which each of the world's countries has sovereignty over its borders and internal activities, was inadequate (Fidler 2004). This was because China failed to fully and accurately disclose information to the WHO about the initial development and then spread of SARS within its borders. In this sense, China's activities impacted widely on the global community. Had the SARS virus been notified to the WHO, and measures taken to prevent its spread when first identified, the estimated US$10–30 billion global costs of the outbreak could have been avoided. The WHO has since worked to forge an international agreement among member countries to act swiftly, honestly and openly in reporting cases of unusual or previously unknown illnesses and disease patterns.

Climate change is another area posing challenges for global as well as national governance. Climate and environmental conditions have long been a health concern, with impacts on availability of clean water, arable land and on living conditions. In some parts of the world, particularly developing regions such as South Asia and China, extreme weather conditions and flooding cause thousands of deaths every year; in Africa and elsewhere droughts routinely take lives. Such conditions also raise the incidence of mental health problems and stress disorders (Ahern et al. 2005). Temperatures around the world have been increasing since the 1970s or so and, by the end of the twenty-first century, are likely to increase by an additional 1.4–5.8 degrees celsius (Intergovernmental Panel on Climate Change 2001).

Climate change, caused by 'greenhouse gas' or carbon emissions, means that extreme weather events are becoming more common. Climate change is also associated with rising sea levels and changes in biodiversity. The public health impacts are likely to be wide ranging. A significant proportion of the world's population living in low lying and coastal areas could be displaced, creating pressure on surrounding areas. Food sources in many already malnourished and poor parts of the world could be affected, while various vector-borne diseases, such as malaria, could spread into areas not previously at risk (Hales et al. 2002; Haines et al. 2006). The transmission season in affected areas could also increase (Tanser et al. 2003). The impacts of climate change are likely to be more serious in the developing world, which has fewer resources to draw upon than the developed world (for instance, to combat vector-borne disease or move people from low-lying areas). However, many developed western countries have also experienced extreme weather events such as Hurricane Katrina which swept over New Orleans and surrounding areas of the

United States in 2005. Nonetheless, global health inequalities are likely to widen as a consequence of climate change.

Countering climate change is an international responsibility but individual country strategies diverge. For example, the United States, which produces around 30 per cent of global carbon emissions, has an obligation to substantially reduce these (World Resources Institute 2006). However, it has refused to date to ratify the 1997 international Kyoto Protocol agreement to reduce emissions. While the federal government has established various goals to reduce greenhouse gas emissions, it stopped short of requiring reductions by law. This is due to a predominant, arguably neoliberal, political view that government should refrain from doing so and that reductions should be voluntary. In something of a 'bottom up' reaction, several US states have mandated emission reductions and large businesses have also acted to reduce their greenhouse gas contributions (Selin and VanDeveer 2007).

The British government, by contrast, played an important role in negotiating and supporting the Kyoto agreement. It continues to be a strong advocate in the international arena for collective action on climate change. Its approach involves supporting development of a European Union emissions trading scheme. In domestic terms, initiatives include legislating to reduce carbon emissions to pre-1990 levels and reporting annually to parliament on progress. Other initiatives have seen new funding for renewable energy sources, improved energy efficiency, and for increased use of alternative fuels (Secretary of State for the Environment, Food and Rural Affairs 2006). A climate change bill, introduced in 2007, enshrined a set of targets for emission reductions, empowered the government to achieve these, and aimed to strengthen the institutional framework for tackling climate change.

Of course, there is a need for greater development and use of public transport, and for policies that contain urban sprawl, promote the conversion of motor vehicles from being powered by petrol to alternative fuels, as the British government is doing, and reduce the distances people commute to work. While such changes could aid the fight against global warming, research also suggests that reductions in air pollution could reduce related deaths in the United States by around 3700–4600 annually (Jacobson et al. 2005). Meanwhile, at an international level:

> Transport is projected to have the fastest proportional growth in greenhouse gas emissions of any sector from 1990–2020, and

there are direct connections with urban air pollution (around 800,000 deaths per year globally), road traffic accidents (1.2 million deaths per year), and physical inactivity (1.9 million deaths a year). There are therefore potentially major synergies in terms of reduced greenhouse gas emissions and direct health benefits from sustainable transport systems that make more use of public transport, walking, and cycling, especially in rapidly developing countries such as China and India.

(Haines et al. 2006: 2108)

Many other issues of concern to public health have potential to stem the pace of climate change. Approximately half the world's population cook over fires, and most of the world's population growth is occurring in developing countries where such cooking and heating methods predominate. More efficient systems, such as cookers powered by sustainable electricity sources, would bring health and economic advantages (Kammen 1995; Haines et al. 2006). The fact that agriculture (especially livestock production) contributes around one-fifth of greenhouse (methane) gas emissions, is also of concern, particularly given increasing consumption of meat per capita. The global average for meat consumption per day is 100 grams, with a ten-fold difference between the highest and lowest consuming countries. An average reduction to 90 grams, with no more than 50 grams being red meat, would bring significant greenhouse gas reductions. It would also reduce the incidence of heart disease, various cancers and obesity (McMichael et al. 2007).

Health inequalities

Health inequalities are of increasing concern to domestic governments. They are also on the international policy agenda as globalization has often been associated with widening inequalities between developed and developing countries (Wermuth 2003). Driving the interest in inequality has been the rapid growth of research evidence from a range of countries that shows that socioeconomic status and other related factors determine how long people live. The consistent pattern is that poorer people have shorter life expectancy and are more likely to suffer from ill health and disease.

The concern for inequality was propelled by the WHO Alma Ata declaration. The first government to investigate the issue was Britain's which commissioned the 'Black Report' of 1980 (Department of Health and Social Security 1980). This highlighted the differences in life expectancy between socioeconomic groups and argued these be reduced by focusing on the 'social determinants' of health; by improving access of disadvantaged people to education, housing, social welfare and health services.

The Black Report arrived at a time of neoliberalism, when Margaret Thatcher was British Prime Minister, and so had minimal impact. This was because the explanations for inequality that the Black Report raised were open to interpretation. It suggested, for instance, that inequalities might be the result of cultural and behavioural factors; that behaviours causing poor health were embedded in social structures and therefore difficult for people to avoid (Department of Health and Social Security 1980). However, as Macintyre later noted, a 'hard' or neoliberal perspective would dismiss this explanation as health damaging behaviours are 'freely chosen' by individuals and not the responsibility of government (Macintyre 1997).

The Black Report did, however, stimulate interest in social determinants of health, as well as inquiries into inequality in countries such as Sweden and the Netherlands. In Britain, the findings from epidemiological studies confirmed the inequalities in health between social classes and pointed again to social factors and structures playing an important role in perpetuating these (Marmot et al. 1991). Elsewhere, studies showed that neoliberal policies, if anything, contributed to widening inequalities within and between countries (Mackenbach and Bakker 2003; Blakely et al. 2005; Navarro 2007).

Since the new millennium, attention to inequality at the international level has been growing. This has been partly driven by data. For example, citizens of the 30 developed world OECD member countries can expect to live around a decade longer on average (around 78 years) than those in non-member countries (around 68 years). The OECD countries have lower infant mortality rates (11 compared with 56 per thousand), and lower HIV prevalence (0.3 per cent compared with 1.1 per cent; UNAIDS 2006; OECD 2007).

International attention on inequality has also been propelled by a changing global focus in keeping with a pendulum swing in the late 1990s away from neoliberalism and toward concern for human development and social democracy. Such concern is represented in the development of the United Nations Millennium Development Goals (MDGs), four of which directly relate to health (see Box 6.2). The MDGs highlighted the new agenda with their attention to partnering the developing world and improving its social and health outcomes, although questions remain over whether the MDGs will

---

Box 6.2: UN Millennium Development Goals

1. eradicate extreme poverty and hunger
2. achieve universal primary education
3. promote gender equality and empower women
4. reduce child mortality
5. improve maternal health
6. combat HIV/AIDS, malaria and other diseases
7. ensure environmental sustainability
8. develop global partnerships for development

---

be achievable by the 2015 target date set by the UN (United Nations Development Programme 2007).

The new millennium has also seen a renewed vigour within the WHO and elsewhere. As with the Black Report, the health for all agenda had been largely sidelined by neoliberalism and the quest for market-oriented health system reform being promoted by agencies such as the World Bank and OECD (Walt and Buse 2006). Social determinants of health is now a central WHO theme. A series of resulting publications has outlined the major causes of inequality and disease. As illustrated in Table 6.2, many of these could be addressed by policy adjustments such as economic reform or improving the availability of healthier foods.

In 2004, the WHO appointed a Commission on Social Determinants of Health. A 2007 Commission publication was underpinned by an analysis of the political variables that influence power relationships within societies. These, the Commission noted, had been lacking in previous WHO work. The Commission argued that social position (where people are in society, which affects health status) was reinforced by stratification (the class and other systems that structure society). To counter this, the Commission proposed a framework for action including tackling structural determinants within society (economic adjustment, improved social services such as housing, education and welfare, and reductions in income inequality); developing and promoting intersectoral policy-making; and engendering community participation in developing policies to address social determinants of health (Commission on Social Determinants of Health 2007; 2008).

Of course, there are strong philosophical and practical arguments to support the WHO's concerns (Woodward and Kawachi 2000;

Table 6.2 Social determinants of health

The social gradient	People further down the ladder run twice the risk of serious illness and premature death than those at the top
Stress	Social and psychological circumstances, such as isolation, insecurity and lack of control over work and home life, can cause long-term stress which raises risks of heart disease, diabetes, depression and aggression
Early life	Poor circumstances during pregnancy can lead to suboptimal foetal development which is linked to health risks in later life
Social exclusion	Poverty, deprivation and social exclusion impact on health and social development and can cause premature death. Such conditions are particularly harmful to children and older people (in the US almost 30 per cent of children live in poor households)
Work	Workplace stress increases the risk of heart and other diseases
Unemployment	Higher rates of unemployment and job insecurity are associated with higher rates of illness and premature death
Social support and cohesion	People with less social support and integration are more likely to suffer mental and physical health problems. Societies with high income inequality have less social cohesion and more violent crime
Addiction	Social deprivation and disadvantage are associated with alcohol and drug use, while addiction also leads to downward social mobility
Food	Good diet is pivotal to health and well-being. Access to good affordable food influences diet more than health education
Transport	Cycling, walking and public transport promote health by reducing fatal accidents and air pollution and increasing social contact

Source: Adapted from Wilkinson and Marmot (2003).

Hausman et al. 2002), as well as a range of research. For example, Navarro and Shi found that countries with political commitment to redistributive economic and social policies, as well as to full employment, were generally more successful in improving population health (Navarro and Shi 2001). The implication is that politics and policy do matter and that social democratic governance is better for health. Similarly, there are multiple studies that look at the impact of economic and social inequality on health outcomes (many are summarized in Marmot and Richardson 2005; Wilkinson 2005). One such study by Pickett and Wilkinson, that compared 23 developed countries as well as all US states, found no association between child well-being and average income. However, what was found was that:

> health and safety and behaviours and risks were significantly worse in more unequal countries. Infant mortality and rates of low birth weight were higher in countries with higher levels of income inequality, as were rates of teenage pregnancy, rates of overweight children, and the proportion of children who reported having been bullied.
>
> (Pickett and Wilkinson 2007: 1083)

The study also found income inequality to be related to lower mathematics scores, fewer young people being in further education and a lower proportion of young people who find their 'peers are kind' (Pickett and Wilkinson 2007). Research also shows that an investment in health has benefits for economic development (Suhrcke et al. 2007).

National governments have pursued various initiatives to reduce inequalities. In Britain, the New Labour government set in train a focus on reducing inequalities, but subsequent policy changes meant variable progress. New Labour appointed a dedicated Minister for Public Health who, propelled by the Acheson Report into inequality (Acheson 1998), announced that inequalities were unacceptable. The government's view was that reducing inequalities required a cross-government agenda and partnerships at all levels of society aimed at improving socioeconomic and environmental conditions (Griffiths and Hunter 2007: 1).

A wide range of 'area based' initiatives followed. In the health field specifically, the government created some 26 Health Action Zones (HAZs). These were partnerships between the NHS, local authorities and business and community groups intended to address local inequalities and improve health. The HAZs covered around one third of the British population and had an extensive reach (Bauld and Judge 2002). They spent around one fifth of their activities focusing on the core determinants of health including improving education and housing services. The remainder was dedicated to health and social services delivery, and developing various programmes in areas such as smoking cessation, sexual health and exercise and nutrition (Asthana and Halliday 2006: 94).

However, HAZs were never adequately funded. Furthermore, they were short lived in that, by 1999, the government had eased back from its commitment to inequalities and was placing emphasis on individual responsibility and use of targets to drive policy objectives (Department of Health 2000a). Policy changes in 2002 then saw PCTs given responsibility for local health services and, along with this, much of the work of HAZs (Asthana and Halliday 2006: 95). As such, a key challenge is the integration of public health into the everyday work of primary care trusts (Hill et al. 2007).

Meanwhile, the British government's favoured policy of setting targets for policy and service delivery, including for reducing inequalities, has had a tendency to perpetuate 'silo' management, where government departments and agencies work to achieve their own objectives at the expense of developing collaborative arrangements (Bogdanor 2005). Thus, while multiple agencies outside of (but also including) the NHS have been charged with inequality reduction, it has been difficult to tell whether the non-health actors are having an impact on health outcomes. Finally, while many of the non-health initiatives produced improvements in areas such as education, employment, housing and poverty, there has been no significant change in overall socioeconomic inequality (Asthana and Halliday 2006: 67; Pickett and Wilkinson 2007). Britain has a rising prevalence of obesity, alcohol consumption, chronic liver disease and cirrhosis, and the highest rate of teenage pregnancy among the 15 European Union member countries (Department of Health 2007). One of the reasons for the sustained inequalities and poor health outcomes may be New Labour's application of neoliberal market-oriented policies. It has favoured ideas of economic self-reliance as the means to protection from poverty and social exclusion, and sought explicitly to inject competition and private sector delivery into the NHS (see Chapter 7).

Reducing inequalities has been a focus of New Zealand health policy since the late 1990s. The first initiatives were introduced by the then National-led centre-right government (1990–1999; Creech 1999). At that point data showed that Maori and Pacific people, in particular, could expect to live around a decade shorter than average. The 1999 election, which produced a centre-left Labour coalition government, brought inequalities to the centre of public policy. Like Britain, the approach has been cross-government. Market-based rentals for public housing were reversed, welfare benefits increased, and considerable effort has been put into bolstering employment and training. Reducing inequalities is the overriding goal of the government's New Zealand Health Strategy and so all health care providers in receipt of public money must describe their plans for this (King 2000). As discussed in Chapter 2, the government has continued to drive the health system with firm contractual targets and financial and other penalties for failure to deliver on these. In this sense, it has used neoliberal methods to tackle inequalities. This has meant providers have been focused on producing data that so that inequalities can be tracked. It also means they have attempted to ensure equal access to services and to eradicate 'institutionalized' practices, such as racism, that perpetuate inequalities (Signal et al. 2007). In many cases, organizations such as DHBs and PHOs have extended services into deprived communities.

The government's Primary Health Care Strategy has provided considerable new funding (around 6–7 percent per annum addition to the health budget) to reduce primary care co-payments which are a significant access barrier (King 2001). This said, primary care providers serving the most deprived communities remain underfunded under the government's funding formula and so patient charges continue (Gauld 2008b). It was intended that both DHBs and PHOs would link with other sectors, such as local government and education, with the aim of reducing inequality and improving public health. However, in a tight funding environment, few such links have emerged. A 2007 study suggested that the government's efforts may be making a difference. From around 1996 the gap in life expectancy between different ethnic and socioeconomic groups appeared to have stabilized and could have begun to decline (Blakely et al. 2007).

Numerous studies and government reports have highlighted the inequalities within US society and the impact these have on health care and outcomes (Institute of Medicine 2003). The US government's 1998 *Healthy People 2010* report noted that African Americans, American Indians and Hispanics have considerably higher rates of infant mortality, heart disease and death from cancers and chronic diseases. They are significantly more likely to not be insured, not to have a regular health care provider and to use emergency services for health care. They are also more likely to receive poorer quality care (US Department of Health and Human Services 1998). Yet, in contrast with Britain and New Zealand, and in keeping with its federal structure, development of inequality (or 'minority') policy in the US has been slow and variable.

At the federal government level, work commissioned during

President Ronald Reagan's tenure led to the creation of the Office of Minority Health. In 2000, President Bill Clinton signed the Health Disparities Research and Education Act. This raised the profile of health inequalities and transformed the Office of Minority Health into the Center for Minority Health and Health Disparities which coordinates country-wide research and training. As a result, many US states now have an office dedicated to minority health (Gamble and Stone 2006). Most of the practical initiatives aimed at reducing disparities have emerged at the state level. However, these have largely revolved around the extension of insurance coverage to previously uninsured groups who, as noted, tend disproportionately to be minorities. Furthermore, only a small number of states have actively sought to improve minority health. To expand coverage, Massachusetts has subsidized premiums for those with incomes below 300 per cent of the federal poverty level. Washington's health insurance law mandates an outreach and education programme to enrol children and focus on groups with the highest rates of uninsurance. In Pennsylvania, a Center for Health Careers has been established to promote diversity and cultural competency among health care professionals. Some states have also permitted data sharing among state agencies to help identify the uninsured and enrol them in public health insurance programmes (Smedley 2008).

Chronic diseases

The term 'chronic disease' is used to describe a range of conditions such as heart disease, stroke, cancers, respiratory illnesses and diabetes that pose a considerable global challenge. Chronic diseases tend to emerge in middle age and are the result of prior unhealthy behaviours and consumption patterns. They are the world's leading cause of death and responsible for around 60 per cent of all deaths. Heart disease represents around 30 per cent of global deaths, cancers around 13 per cent, respiratory diseases seven per cent and diabetes two per cent (Horton 2005). In 2005, 35 million people died from chronic diseases. Half of these people were under 70 years of age and half were women. The burden of chronic disease is weighted toward the developing world, with around 80 per cent of deaths in low and middle income countries. Compared with higher income countries, these deaths are more likely to occur among younger people. Furthermore, deaths from some chronic illnesses, such as heart disease, have declined since the 1960s in many developed countries, but contined to increase in most developing countries (Leeder et al.

2004). The major risk factors for chronic disease are smoking, lack of exercise, poor nutrition and physical inactivity (see www.who.int/chp/en) all of which are modifiable (Quam et al. 2006).

Policy makers are concerned about chronic diseases for various reasons. Foremost is that the increase in chronic diseases is projected to continue. As noted, the developing world faces particular challenges in this respect, especially with heart disease where rates are predicted to increase between 1990 and 2020 by 120 per cent for women and 137 per cent for men (Leeder et al. 2004). The prevalence of diabetes is projected to increase from 2.8 per cent of the global population in 2000 to 6.5 per cent in 2030 although this prediction does not account for increases in childhood and adult obestity which will impact on type 2 diabetes rates. Cancers, also, have continued to increase with estimates of a 19 per cent increase between 1990 and 2000 (Yach et al. 2006). The increase of people who are overweight or obese is a particular concern due to the association with other chronic diseases especially type 2 diabetes, hypertension, strokes, heart disease and respiratory problems. Research has also shown that increasing body mass is associated with a significant increase in the risk of a range of cancers (Reeves et al. 2007). In North America, the proportion of people who were obese increased from 15 per cent of the population in 1976–1980 to 32.9 per cent in 2003–2004 (see http://www.cdc.gov/nccdphp/dnpa/obesity/index.htm).

North America is not alone as the proportion of obese people in many countries continues to grow. Across many Asian countries, for instance, the proportions of the population presently obese remain comparatively small but are increasing, while the numbers of overweight people are similar to many developed western countries. Furthermore, levels of diabetes are also comparable and there is evidence that Asian people develop diabetes with a lesser degree of obesity and at younger ages. The rapid economic growth and urbanization in China and India, and increase in childhood obesity, are of particular concern (Yoon et al. 2006).

Another concern is that the incidence of chronic disease is contributing to the growing costs of health care provision. As noted, chronic disease tends to favour poorer and deprived populations and so perpetuates inequalities both within and between countries (Beaglehole and Yach 2003). The less well off are more prone to illness and chronic disease ensures that they stay poor. Finally, the causes of many chronic diseases, while well known, seem particularly difficult to counter. This is because they are often the result of a complex array of factors and situations. These include socioeconomic circumstance and societal structures and cultures that influence people's behaviours, as well as the limited availability of and access to resources that have the potential to improve public health.

Reflecting the complexity, there are a wide range of suggestions for combatting chronic disease. Increasingly, these are being taken up by international organizations such as the WHO and the 'Clinton Global Initiative' (led by former US President Bill Clinton), concerned about addressing the chronic disease 'epidemic'. Such organizations reflect the sentiments of national governments and also seek to influence their policy agendas as well as the activities of business. The Clinton initiative, for example, is working to partner with multinational food manufacturers (such as PepsiCo), the pharmaceutical industry, and many non-government agencies to develop innovative ways of reducing chronic disease (Quam et al. 2006).

Many countries have banned tobacco advertising and smoking in public places including bars and restaurants, increased tobacco taxes and funded smoking cessation programmes. Some, such as Denmark and Switzerland, have banned the use of trans fats. Short of countrywide bans, cities such as Calgary and New York have banned the use of these fats in restaurants. There are growing calls that urban design should facilitate walking and that physical movement should be promoted by all sectors within society: schools, workplaces, and by cities and governments (Lean et al. 2006). Moreover, there are calls that access to unhealthy foods and drinks should be limited and backed by sustained policies (such as bans within schools), that the food supply chain should be regulated to make healthy choices easier, that marketing of high energy foods and drinks to children should be restricted and even banned, and that the benefits of healthy eating and physical activity should be routinely promoted (Swinburne et al. 2004; James et al. 2007).

Health promotion has a particularly important role to play in the context of chronic disease, with all sorts of new initiatives and approaches emerging. These range from attempts to develop healthy communities through community engagement projects that network different organizations and groups, through to the use of text messages and the Internet which have been found to assist individuals working to change their health behaviours (Cook et al. 2007).

There has been a resurgence of targets and goals for reducing chronic disease and tackling the contributing factors. Unlike targets for financial performance or quality improvement, it is difficult to apply neoliberal concepts to chronic disease improvement. Instead, governments have recognized that this is an area that demands coordinated and community-oriented government strategies. Often targets and goals, such as enrolling a specific number of people at risk of chronic disease in a health promotion programme, are components of such strategies.

For example, Sweden's National Public Health Policy includes goals to increase physical activity and nutrition, while Finland has a 'three-pronged' strategy to reduce type 2 diabetes. Both Denmark and France aim to reduce the incidence of obesity. The French target is for a 20 per cent reduction in adult obesity (Allin et al. 2004). Britain's GBP373 million Healthy Weight, Healthy Lives strategy aims by 2011, through the national school curriculum, to educate children about healthy cooking and a healthy diet. By 2012, a walking campaign intends for one third of people to walk an additional 1000 steps a day. There are also incentives for employers to promote healthy living and exercise (Department of Health 2008a). The New Zealand Health Strategy underpins the activities of all government-funded service providers. It places a strong emphasis on chronic disease reduction through health promotion and coordinated service delivery for identified 'at risk' groups and individuals (King 2000). Annual reports detail progress in implementing the New Zealand Health Strategy goals (for example, Ministry of Health 2006). The US also has an approach based around health promotion and collaboration concepts, with federal government working closely with various states to reduce obesity. Initiatives include 'multi-sector' partnerships involving selected communities, joint ventures between state public health departments and health maintenance organizations aimed at influencing the health behaviours of children and young people, and the application of social marketing approaches (Centers for Disease Control 2008).

CONCLUSION

This chapter overviewed key issues in public health. It looked at changing ideas about health determinants and at concepts of 'new public health' that are behind the present health policies of many governments and the international community. The chapter discussed contemporary public health concerns and the many influences on the public health agenda today, including increasing research evidence and the global and national impacts of public health issues.

The swing toward social democracy in Britain, New Zealand and a range of other countries has corresponded with an emphasis on reducing inequalities and pursuit of components of a new public health agenda. Britain and New Zealand have political systems that permit national approaches, although Britain failed to provide adequate support for implementing inequalities policy (Exworthy et al. 2002), and subsequently moved to neoliberal designs. New Zealand has been closest to having a consistent focus on public health issues, requiring that local planning boards and primary care providers pursue public health goals and targets. In contrast, in the US some states have implemented measures to tackle inequalities and chronic disease, but these have been mostly limited to extending service access in an insurance driven system.

Whether initiatives such as those outlined in this chapter can satisfy the tremendous demands on the public health agenda is questionable. The WHO argues that more needs to be done to alter societal structures. Looking at historical lessons, implementation of the comparatively uncontentious WHO primary care agenda has been slow (Rifkin and Walt 1986; World Health Organization 2008). As such, it might be little surprise that no government has yet announced reforms based on the WHO Commission on Social Determinants of Health framework. While important in public health terms, reforming socioeconomic structures (meaning alterations to tax systems, the labour market, and so forth) could be difficult in political terms to achieve.

Issues such as climate change throw into stark relief the challenges facing both the developing and developed world. Countries such as the US need to do more to reduce their greenhouse gas emission and consumption patterns, to set an example and demonstrate that they are leading the way. The US case, as outlined in this chapter, illustrates how a 'hands off', or neoliberal, approach could fail to provide the leadership needed for tackling climate change. The British approach, by contrast, is underpinned by social democratic concerns for an international collaborative effort. Whether it and others, such as the various non-government actors, can provide for the changes required to act on public health issues will continue to be an important question.

QUESTIONS FOR FURTHER DISCUSSION

1. What are the aims of public health and what are some of the main determinants of health?
2. Why is public health important to health policy today?

3. What are the key public health issues facing developed world governments, and what should be done about these?
4. Would a neoliberal or a social democratic agenda be more likely to promote public health?

7

THE PRIVATE SECTOR

This chapter explores:

- The role of the private sector in health care and systems
- How this role differs across countries and issues
- How and why governments have reintroduced 'competition and choice' into their health systems

INTRODUCTION

The private sector plays an important role in virtually every one of the world's health systems. Most countries feature a combination of public and private funding and service provision. In some countries, such as the United States, private funding and service providers dominate the delivery of health care and there is strong political and societal support for such arrangements. In other countries, including Canada, Britain, Australia and many European Union members, the private sector plays an important but significantly smaller role than that of the public sector. In health systems where the state dominates, the private sector's contribution may be in providing particular services.

The private sector, however, is considerably broader than a simple contributor to the delivery of health services. Private business dominates the design and manufacture of pharmaceuticals of which the government in many countries is a major purchaser. Governments, of course, also regulate drugs. Private interests are behind the medical devices industry which supplies equipment to assist with surgical procedures and other treatments. Some governments actively seek private funding to build public hospitals and other facilities.

Debates over the role and extent of private involvement in health systems are ongoing. In the neoliberal era, governments explicitly sought to boost private involvement in the delivery of publicly-funded health care. They aimed to both reduce the 'burden' on the state, while attempting to create a private sector that would compete with public service providers. There remains a lack of clarity over a series of private sector issues including what its optimal role in a health system should be, whether the private sector delivers better and more cost effective services, and whether the pursuit of competition and patient choice is in the public's best interest. Despite this, there has been a recent push in some countries to reintroduce elements of the neoliberal market model by stimulating private delivery of publicly-funded services.

This chapter overviews the role of the private sector in health systems. The opening section looks at how the private sector is involved in different health systems and components of service delivery. This section also outlines debates around whether government should be the dominant player in health care and considers evidence of private sector performance. Second, the chapter discusses the re-emergence of government policies designed to promote private market concepts of competition and choice. The case of Britain is highlighted as its government has pushed farther in these directions than others, but other countries are also discussed. The conclusion considers whether policies to boost competition and private services have the potential to improve health systems.

PRIVATE SECTOR INVOLVEMENT IN HEALTH SYSTEMS

As noted in Chapter 2, there are differing ways of funding and organizing health care. The mix that most countries feature invariably includes a private component. There is no recognized proportion of a health system that it is unequivocally believed should be provided for via private means, nor is there agreement over which services or components of a health system are amenable to private provision. What there is are variations across countries that reflect historical system development, the type of health system, and political preferences around the role of the public sector (Scott 2001; Blank and Burau 2004; Gauld 2005a). Some countries, such as Britain, have a tradition of public sector dominance and a strong philosophical belief that health care ought to be universally accessible and without a cost barrier to individual patients. Other countries, such as the US, are driven by notions of individualism, self-reliance and competition. Their health funding arrangements and systems are underpinned by the idea that private business should dominate service provision, that patients should have choice among providers, and that it should not be a government responsibility to provide for each and every health care need.

Public-private funding split

One measure that provides a rough insight into the extent of the private sector is the basic split between public and private sources of total funding. Figure 7.1 illustrates this split across OECD countries. The table shows that public funding is the dominant source, but that there are some outliers such as the United States. However, the data in Figure 7.1 do not show what private funding contributes to in individual countries, nor how the public and private sectors interface. For example, in Canada the full range of public services carry no charges, but most of these 'public' services are delivered by private providers. General practitioners, working out of private facilities, receive a full government payment per patient. Hospital specialists providing publicly-funded care are mostly private practitioners, paid by the government on a fee-for-service basis, yet the hospitals that they practise in are all public. Services that are not covered by public insurance such as podiatry, dentistry and optometry, receive no subsidy. Funding for these via private insurance and personal payments accounts for much of the Canadian private expenditure (Kenny and Chafe 2007). Many Canadian businesses provide private health insurance as part of the employment benefit package, in this way presenting themselves to prospective employees as an employer of choice. Data show that employer-provided insurance is not uncommon and that this is one reason why, in many countries, private funding of health care has been increasing at well above the general inflation rate (Munn and Wozniak 2007). Governments, of course, often provide tax incentives for employers to offer such insurance.

Interestingly, the Canada Health Act of 1984, which enshrined a set of principles for the Canadian health system, outlawed private insurance for services covered by public health insurance. This implies a state commitment to providing a wide range of services for the entire Canadian population, but also means that there is no market for private specialists and there are very few geniunely private

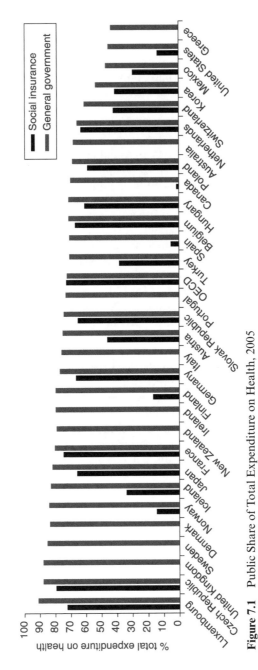

Figure 7.1 Public Share of Total Expenditure on Health, 2005

Source: OECD (2007).

practitioners in Canada. It also means that people requiring non-urgent treatments have no alternative but to wait for treatment in public hospitals. Those willing or able to pay and wanting to circumvent waiting lists, perhaps only a fraction of the Canadian population, have to go abroad for service.

The British NHS features more private involvement than is apparent from Figure 7.1. Like Canada and many other countries, the NHS is predominantly tax-funded. Yet its general practitioners are largely private contractors in receipt of public money. Around 30 per cent of the NHS budget is spent on privately-provided pharmaceuticals, medical devices and other equipment. Furthermore, the NHS has long purchased the services of private specialists to perform a small proportion of non-urgent procedures (Timmins 2005b). As discussed later in this chapter, government policies introduced since 2000 mean the NHS is increasingly buying services from private surgical service providers. In sum, the NHS is a system in which funding is mostly public, but as with other countries much public funding goes to private sources.

New Zealand has similarities to the NHS case. While services are mostly public and tax-funded, the private sector plays an important role. General practitioners are all private, but receive substantial government funding. Private hospitals do not deliver emergency care. However, like Britain and Canada, New Zealand's public hospitals have waiting lists for elective procedures. The private sector, therefore, fills an important role in providing swift access to those with insurance or ability to pay. The public sector does, on occasion, purchase elective procedures from private hospitals for public patients. In general, such procedures are performed by specialists who hold appointments in public hospitals, but also maintain a private practice where they generate substantially more income than from their salaried public positions. This has often led to charges that public waiting lists benefit such practitioners; that they should not be permitted to straddle both the public and private sectors. Substantial subsidies are also provided for prescribed pharmaceuticals, as discussed below, and most laboratory tests are performed by private contractors. The relative role of the private sector in New Zealand has varied over time. As discussed in Chapter 2, in the 1990s era of neoliberalism, there were attempts to increase private provision of elective and other services. Since 1999, with the election of a social democratic government, emphasis has been on building public sector funding and capacity. That said, under pressure to curtail expenditure, local DHBs are increasingly seeking private sector solutions.

An interesting case is that of South Korea where public funding is around 53 per cent of the total. Funding is split in various ways. The bulk of public funding is from a single national social insurance agency, which is a division of the government Ministry of Health. Social insurance pays for around 44 per cent of the costs of hospital and primary care. A government funded Medicaid scheme pays for the care of those not covered by social insurance. Although social insurance is 'universal', in that all working South Koreans and their dependents are covered, and for a relatively comprehensive range of services, co-payments are substantial amounting to around 37 per cent of all private funding in the system. Private insurance picks up the remainder. The high co-payments pose a significant access barrier for many and undermine the attempt, with social insurance, to provide equity. While the funding system is government adminis-tered and dominated, service provision is largely private. Indeed, less than 10 per cent of beds are in public hospitals, but these tend to treat more Medicaid patients and provide cheaper services which are not covered by social insurance. There is fierce competition among service providers, including between the public and private sectors. This is because patients have complete freedom to choose among providers, as there is no gatekeeping within the system, but also as patients bring social insurance payments and are therefore the chief source of income (Kwon 2005).

Several of the European Union countries listed in Figure 7.1 feature social insurance. While such funding is categorized as public, the implications for the private sector are considerable. Social insur-ance, as noted in Chapter 2, is sometimes provided by private com-panies and so there is often a large private insurance industry. Social insurance also requires payments from both private employers and employees. The trade off is usually that there is compensation by way of tax relief. Naturally, when government makes a decision to change the rules or organization of social insurance, this will have implica-tions for private business. This was the case in the Netherlands with its insurance reforms of 2006 which brought together former social and private insurance arrangements into one single mandatory scheme, regulated under private law. The reforms led to concerns among private employers and insurers that their share of health insurance funding could eventually increase by up to 30 per cent (van Ginneken 2006).

Alongside social insurance providers will often also be a private health insurance industry offering a range of packages, from add-itional to full coverage. The extent of private insurance coverage

differs widely between countries (see Figure 7.2). In some, such
as the US and the Netherlands, private insurance is the primary
source of health care funding. As noted, this is compulsory in the
Netherlands but not the US. In most OECD countries, private insurance contributes to part of the funding mix, with different roles in
different systems (OECD 2007). This mix of public and private
insurance means many countries are able to achieve full insurance
coverage for their populations. Germany, for example, has around
250 social insurance providers, and 49 private health insurers. The

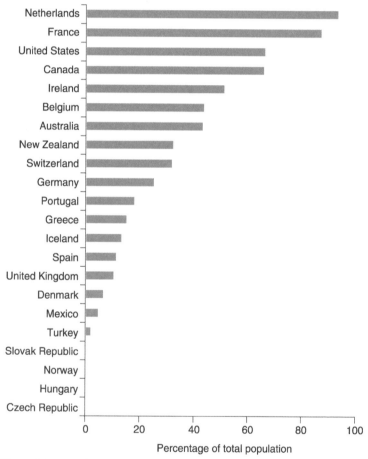

Figure 7.2   Population covered by private health insurance, 2005
Source: OECD (2007).

private providers cater to high-income Germans who opt-out of social insurance (OECD 2007). As the capacity for social insurance in Germany to provide comprehensive benefits has come under pressure, the uptake of private insurance has gradually increased (Furstenbuerg et al. 2007). Around 87 per cent of French residents have 'complementary' private insurance to fund service copayments that the social security system does not cover. Sixty-six per cent of Canadians have 'supplementary' private insurance to fund services not reimbursed by government funding. Then there are countries with 'duplicate' insurance markets, such as Ireland, Australia and New Zealand. Here, private insurance facilitates timely access for those with coverage to privately-provided services that they would otherwise have to wait for in the public sector.

Pharmaceuticals

Figure 7.3 shows that OECD countries spend a considerable amount of money on privately manufactured pharmaceuticals when measured as a percentage of GDP. Pharmaceuticals are an interesting case as no government in the world is involved in their manufacture, and so governments and the public are entirely reliant on the private sector for supply. Some developing world governments actively encourage their local generics industry in order to increase drug availability, and turn a blind eye when branded drug patents are infringed, much to the ire of the international pharmaceutical industry. While some of the OECD countries listed in Figure 7.3 provide minimal or no subsidies for pharmaceuticals, many provide substantial public funding to reduce direct patient costs. This is reflected in the percentage of the government budget spent on pharmaceuticals. At the top end is the Slovak Republic where almost 30 per cent of government expenditure is on drugs with Poland (27 per cent) and South Korea (26 per cent) close behind. Governments with limited direct pharmaceutical expenditure include Norway (8 per cent), Luxembourg, (8.4 per cent) and Denmark (9.8 per cent; OECD 2008). On average, OECD country governments fund 60 per cent of all domestic pharmaceutical expenditure (OECD 2007). All governments are also, of course, deeply involved in regulating the pharmaceutical industry and monitoring drug performance. This includes the safety of drugs but also the behaviour of the industry.

The prices governments and publicly-funded service providers pay for pharmaceuticals vary between countries and are often determined through a process of negotiation. Some countries have an

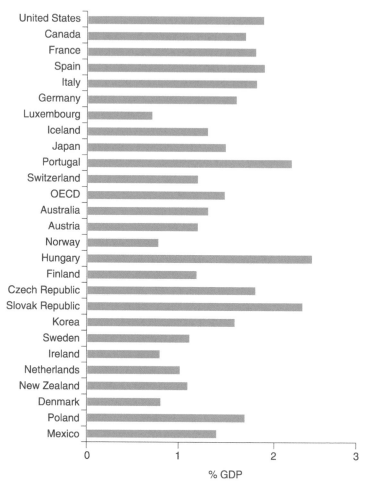

Figure 7.3   Pharmaceutical expenditure as a percentage of GDP, 2005
Source: OECD (2007).

agency specifically dedicated to government-funded pharmaceutical purchasing, much to the ire of the pharmaceutical industry. New Zealand's Pharmaceutical Management Agency (Pharmac) is frequently cited as one of the more successful such examples. Pharmac was created in the neoliberal era of the 1990s and in this period was located at arms' length from central government. It functioned as would a private business, seeking to obtain more product while delivering efficiency gains. Since 1999, Pharmac has been under closer government control and expected to deliver on a range of new social objectives. As such, it now also works to change prescribing behaviours and societal attitudes towards medicines.

Charged with managing the government's schedule of publicly-subsidized drugs, and therefore a 'bulk purchaser' with considerable buying power, Pharmac has used various strategies over the years to drive down pharmaceutical company prices (see Davis 2004). The agency claims it kept government drug expenditure costs and cost growth well below what they might otherwise have been. The pharmaceutical industry, for its part, has long suggested that Pharmac's tactics have denied the New Zealand public access to a range of medicines. At times, the industry has placed considerable pressure on Pharmac. It has taken Pharmac to court over some funding decisions, and launched public campaigns designed to discredit the agency. The industry's concerns have been shared by others. For example, Pharmac decisions around funding of particular medications, such as statins which are known to reduce cholesterol levels and cardiovascular events, have been challenged by the medical profession, researchers, and patient advocacy groups alike (see, for example, Ellis and White 2006). They have been unhappy with Pharmac's preference for funding generics, suggesting in some cases that these are inferior; nor have they condoned the focus on driving down prices paid to pharmaceutical companies for the fact that this has, in some cases, resulted in reduced access to medicines (Martin and Begg 2000; Swinburne et al. 2000). It has not been uncommon for the government to become involved in such cases, and for additional funding to be made available to reinstate a branded drug that may have been removed from the Pharmac funding schedule.

Pharmaceutical distribution and dispensing is often dominated by private providers. In many countries, patients have pharmaceutical prescriptions filled by pharmacists in private practice. Such businesses will be under strict government regulation and they will only be able to dispense authorized medicines. These pharmacists may generate a significant income from the supply of medicines that carry government subsidies. Many countries also feature government-owned pharmacies that work in conjunction with other public institutions such as hospitals and primary care organizations. The pharmaceutical industry, of course, spends enormous sums of money developing and promoting its products and has often been found to have placed profit interests ahead of public safety (Callahan and Wasunna 2006; DeAngelis 2006; Mello and Joffe 2007, Ch. 5).

Most countries, except for the United States and New Zealand, outlaw direct-to-consumer advertising. This means that the industry, unable to directly influence patients, is reliant on trying to influence prescribing behaviour. Research has shown that pharmaceutical companies use various methods for this, including providing gifts to doctors and that, in so doing, they often breach their own code of ethics (McNeill et al. 2006). Companies also sponsor medical conferences. Despite pledges that such sponsorship is not designed to influence prescribing behaviour, evidence suggests that pharmaceutical companies are often consulted about the acceptability of speakers they are sponsoring and so have the potential to influence the messages projected (Moynihan 2008).

Public-private partnerships

The building of partnerships between public and private providers has been increasing since the 1990s, further adding to debates that the private sector has an important role to play. Public-private partnerships have predominantly occurred in the context of the developing world, especially Africa and South Asia (Widdus 2005). They have often been in response to failures of both governments and the private sector to provide services, and failures in general of policies such as those of the World Bank in the neoliberal era that were aimed at promoting private sector solutions (Buse and Harmer 2007).

Public-private partnerships have generally been forged for specific purposes. Most have been around the treatment of neglected diseases such as tuberculosis, malaria and HIV/AIDS. There have also been partnerships aimed at improving access to drugs, including making generics and low-cost branded drugs available specifically for developing countries. The developing world is poorly served by the pharmaceutical industry. Indeed, an analysis of private sector medicines developments showed that only a fraction of new drugs were for diseases that afflict the developing world (Trouiller et al. 2002). Drug development is predominantly aimed at diseases of the wealthy world where governments and individuals are willing and able to pay.

Some public-private partnerships have been focused on providing access to crucial medicines that neither affected populations nor their respective governments are able to fund. As such, they have been designed to bring public and donor funding together with private expertise or pharmaceutical providers who otherwise would have little financial incentive to make products and services available.

Notably, few public-private partnerships have been aimed at broader issues such as health system improvement (Barr 2007). There has been considerable excitement around the fact that many partnerships have produced positive results such as improving disease management and access to medicines; they have often also done so while controlling costs (Karki et al. 2007). Yet the jury remains out about whether public-private partnerships are a panacea. The role of the private sector in particular continues to be questioned, especially its motives, even when efforts have considerable public health benefits. There has been a propensity for private interests to dominate in partnership governance arrangements (Barr 2007; Buse and Harmer 2007). There also remains a need for much more research into costing arrangements and to 'reassess the prevailing [neoliberal] paradigm which presupposes that market-based approaches are necessarily more efficient than public sector ones' (Buse and Harmer 2007: 269).

In a developed-world manifestation of partnership arrangements, some countries have explicitly sought private finance for the building of public health care facilities. An example is Britain's Private Finance Initiative (PFI) which requires that all public service agencies, including NHS hospitals, seek to partner the private sector for funding capital projects. Such partnerships typically involve a 30-year contract. Prior to 1997, almost all NHS investment was funded directly by the government. Since then at least 85 per cent of capital funding has come from private sources under PFI arrangements. Yet initial analysis of such projects suggested that, while improved maintenance standards would most probably result and projects may be more likely to be completed on time, the cost of private finance was likely to surpass that of traditionally-provided public capital due to the higher costs of private borrowing (Sussex 2003). Partnerships have also been formed for development of large national information technology projects, as is the case in Denmark (Vrangbaek 2008).

SHOULD GOVERNMENT DOMINATE HEALTH CARE FUNDING AND PROVISION?

There are strong arguments for a dominant public role in health systems. These include that governments have the capacity to create universal and equitable access to a full range of services by ensuring that costs to individuals are heavily subsidized, meaning that the less well off are able to access expensive and life-saving treatments without concern for cost. Governments are able to make decisions to increase funding levels or extend services where necessary. They are able to pool public money in ways that private insurers cannot do or have no interest in and use this 'monopsony' power to drive down costs such as for the purchase of pharmaceuticals. They also have the potential to deliver services without the administrative costs associated with contracting among competing funders and providers in an unfettered marketplace.

With the world's highest expenditure on health care per capita and as a percentage of GDP, the US – the country closest to having a health system founded on market principles – fails to deliver universal service access. In 2008, approximately 47 million North Americans were without health insurance and so had no guaranteed way to fund health care as a result. Those most affected were on lower incomes or out of work. Insurance coverage has been in decline as the costs to business and individuals increase. This has led to suggestions that the US health system, with its inherent focus on competition and private provision, is fundamentally flawed; that its for-profit institutions provide inferior quality at inflated cost; that administration costs are unnecessarily high (almost double Canada's, for example); and that other countries should look elsewhere for reform lessons (Woolhandler and Himmelstein 2007). Research has even revealed diminishing confidence among North American health care leaders in the idea that competition can drive system improvement (Nichols et al. 2004). As noted elsewhere in this book, the response to market failure in a selection of US states has involved cross-sector bargains between the private insurance industry, employers, state government and the federal Medicare programme to reduce insurance costs and extend coverage. The state of Massachusetts has created an insurance 'exchange' that provides information about price, quality and coverage of all available plans to facilitate comparisons. Owing to the success of the Massachusetts efforts, the federal government has increased its funding allocation to the state to aid further insurance coverage (Long 2008).

Despite the US experience of drastic market failure and state-level rescue efforts, there has been a keen interest in many countries in enhancing the private sector. An initial wave that commenced in the 1980s was driven by neoliberalism as outlined in Chapters 1 and 2. There is evidence that the creation of 'markets' in government-dominated health systems and embracing of private providers during this first wave resulted in some initial increases in private funding sources but that such a shift was shortlived (Oliver 2007). Evidence also suggests that private provision failed to reduce pressure on the public sector, and that where public funding was reduced in favour of private funding this undermined levels of public satisfaction in health systems (Tuohy et al. 2004). New Zealand's surge in the 1990s towards neoliberal market approaches is a prime example. Public hospital waiting lists soared along with hospital funding pressures. Clinical staff morale was undermined and new generic 'managers' experienced considerable difficulty attempting to justify the introduction of patient charges and service cutbacks. The net result was that patient safety was jeopardized (Stent 1998), the public were deeply dissatisfied, and substantial government funding injections were required (Gauld 2001).

The debates around private involvement are wide ranging. Research shows that there are questions around assertions that private providers are more efficient or provide better quality services. A systematic review of existing studies found that there was a lower risk of mortality among dialysis patients in private not-for-profit health centres than in private for-profit organizations, underscoring the notion that a focus on profitability can undermine quality of care (Devereaux et al. 2002). A similar type of study found that the costs of treatment in private for-profit hospitals was higher than in non-profit hospitals again leading to the conclusion that there was no economic rationale to suggest that policy makers should promote private for-profit provision of hospital services (Devereaux et al. 2004). A study of North American Medicare enrollees found that those in non-profit insurance plans received significantly higher quality of care than those in purely for-profit plans (Schneider et al. 2005).

Other studies, however, have fuelled arguments that purely 'public' or government-funded services could do better if they were more like private non-profit organizations. The distinction between 'for-profit' and 'non-profit' private institutions may well be crucial in the context of governments looking to 'private' systems for lessons. In 2002, Feachem et al. compared the performance of the British NHS with that of California's non-profit yet private Kaiser Permanente across a range of available indicators (Feachem et al. 2002). They argued that the two systems had some similarities and so were comparable. However, some commentators suggested the two systems had more differences than similarities, such as the fact that the NHS is universally accessible whereas Kaiser deals with patients enrolled through insurance schemes and is therefore inaccessible to certain groups. Doctors working for Kaiser also tend to do so because of its explicit philosophy of providing 'equitable service' to all those enrolled with it, unlike many other US managed care organizations which are wholly driven by patient ability to pay (Shapiro and Smith 2003).

Feachem et al. found that the costs for service provision in both Kaiser and the NHS were similar to within ten per cent, but that Kaiser's performance was superior. Kaiser patients had better clinical outcomes, shorter service waiting times and fewer inpatient bed stays for preventable illness. The reasons for this, it was asserted, were that Kaiser services were better integrated, with more emphasis on treating patients at the most cost effective level of care. In other words, Kaiser delivered many services in the community that the NHS provided in more expensive hospital settings. Kaiser hospitals were also better managed, and competition, inherent within the US health system, had served to focus the organization on improving its efficiency (Feachem et al. 2002). It is this idea of competition, rooted in neoliberalism, where services with incentives to improve quality and compete with one another for patients and market share, which has been influential in other countries seeking to improve public sector performance.

A subsequent study by Ham et al. found that the NHS provided three and a half times the number of acute bed days as Kaiser, and double that of North American Medicare (government insured) services. Like Feachem et al., this study also concluded that the NHS had much to learn from Kaiser's integrated approach (Ham et al. 2003).

REINTRODUCING 'COMPETITION' AND 'CHOICE'

While the discussions in the preceding sections suggest a lack of unequivocal evidence to support private sector enhancement, studies such as those of the North American Kaiser experience have helped to provide justification for a second wave of health system reforms aimed at boosting the private sector. These reforms, which have often been promoted by governments pursuing social democratic objectives laced with neoliberal policies, have sought to reintroduce competition among service funders and providers and to provide choice for patients.

The British case

As discussed in Chapter 1, neoliberalism led many countries to pursue market designs for their health systems. A classic example was Britain, where the government introduced an 'internal market' in 1991. The initial view of the new Blair government, elected in 1997, was that ideas of markets and competition had been damaging to the NHS. Instead, 'partnership' and 'collaboration' would be emphasized.

However, since 2000, there has been a gradual reintroduction of competition and choice within the NHS. The 2000 NHS Plan, designed to 'modernize' the NHS, made significant new service funding available (a 7.5 per cent increase per annum from 2000 to 2008). Modernization also meant having an open mind with regard to the private sector, particularly given that the government wanted more operations to be performed and the public sector lacked capacity to do so. Accordingly, the Plan, and a succeeding implementation document, suggested NHS purchasers could use spare private sector capacity where public hospitals were unable to provide services in a timely or cost-effective manner that might affect achievement of performance targets, and that a wider range of providers ought to be accessible by NHS patients. Furthermore, patients should be able to choose between service providers – public or private. The idea here was that the NHS would remain the funder, maintaining the social democratic principle of universality, and simply purchase services from various providers. If care remained free at the point of service, then the basic philosophy of the NHS would not be undermined (Timmins 2005a). As noted above, there was also support for public-private partnerships for hospital building projects.

The government began a process of giving better performing hospitals more financial freedom than others, engendering competition for such status. In 2004, the government further moved to increase competition and choice. In primary care, through the commitment of significant additional funding, a radical new pay for performance contract for GPs was introduced which built on a pre-existing but more limited programme. While focused on quality improvement, the new contract explicitly tied financial incentives, an idea borrowed from the private sector, to the achievement of performance targets (Campbell et al. 2007).

In secondary care, the government had, in the late 1990s, created NHS 'treatment centres' designed to increase service delivery capacity for routine non-urgent treatments in the attempt to tackle hospital waiting lists. From 2003, it decided to encourage the establishment of 'independent sector treatment centres' (ISTCs). Like the earlier treatment centres, ISTCs perform routine procedures and diagnostic services on contract to the NHS. However, ISTCs were to be run by private providers, thus creating a provider market to compete with NHS services and facilitating patient choice between public and private providers. By 2007, there were 24 ISTCs being run by seven for-profit companies delivering 10 per cent of NHS non-urgent services. Around a quarter of ISTC staff were on secondment from the NHS posing threats to NHS service sustainability (Ferris 2005; Pollock and Godden 2008).

In 2007, the government announced that it would be allowing private companies to operate NHS general practices, and that it would also be establishing over 150 new primary care health centres, 'many of which will probably be run by private companies' (Salisbury 2008). These centres are to function as polyclinics, with longer opening hours and a wider range of services than traditional general practices. The government continues to introduce new policies to sharpen competition and choice. For example, in 2008, it announced that health care providers, both NHS and private, would be able to advertise their services including waiting times, surgical outcomes and infection rates. Endorsements from former patients, such as celebrities, would be allowed, so long as they were not paid for doing so. The government also announced a GBP600,000 campaign of radio and newspaper advertisements designed to promote the idea of patient choice (Cohen 2008). Lastly, the final report of the 2008 Darzi review endorsed giving individuals control of their own personal NHS health care budgets. Designed to further push providers toward tailoring services to individuals, the policy will be introduced for specific long-term care patients in 2009 (Department of Health 2008).

Competition and choice elsewhere

Competition and choice has also been pursued by several European Union member countries. Denmark, which has a predominantly tax-funded health system, has introduced a series of reforms that have boosted the role of the private sector. Initial reforms of 1993 allowed for patients to receive treatment at any public hospital in the country, thus providing for an element of choice and attempting to stimulate hospitals into providing non-urgent services within a government-set two month timeframe (Strandberg-Larsen et al. 2007).

A 2002 'Welfare and Choice' reform, implemented by a centre-right Liberal-Conservative coalition government, was designed to further stimulate private sector involvement in the delivery of public services. Here, the 'free choice' policy was extended by allowing patients to choose a private provider in Denmark or abroad, fully funded by the government, if treatment could not be publicly provided within two months. Under this arrangement, private providers – local and foreign – would need to have a formal contract with one of the five (previously 14) publicly-funded regional purchasing authorities.

In 2007, the government shortened its treatment target to one month, therefore stimulating additional competition among public hospitals to provide timely service or lose patients to the private sector. Private hospitals were, perhaps naturally, supportive of the new policy directions. Public institutions, for their part, expressed concern that the one month target was too tight. Yet they also suggested that they might be able to improve their performances if the government permitted them to provide 'overtime' services so that operating hours and capacity could be extended. As with Britain, the new competition and choice policy has raised questions over 'dual clinical practice' where physicians work in both public and private institutions; particularly, that higher private sector pay could reduce public sector provider capacity, but also provide incentives for clinicians to encourage public patients into private facilities (Socha and Bech 2007). There have also been concerns that Denmark's choice policies have tended to advantage younger, more mobile, wealthier and healthier people and have been administratively cumbersome (Thomson and Dixon 2006)

The promotion of competition and choice has been similarly evident in the Netherlands. Market-oriented reforms were initially suggested by a government-appointed committee in 1986. While never implemented, incremental changes paved the way for later developments. Thus, in 2006, a centre-right government reformed social insurance with the implementation of a new Health Insurance Act. The new arrangements are designed to curtail rising health expenditure and to introduce more competition among health insurers. The reforms are also designed to extend coverage to the entire population and thus fulfil social democratic goals. Every Dutch citizen is now required to purchase health insurance from a field of private providers who are regulated by the government. Employers also contribute by compensating employees and receive a tax-rebate in return. Insurers must provide a standard set of benefits but can also offer supplementary insurance. To facilitate choice and drive competition, people are annually able to shift their coverage between insurers who compete over premium levels, service, and quality of care offered by contracted health care providers (Enthoven and van de Ven 2007). By 2007, 98.5 per cent of all eligible Dutch people had enrolled. However, as with Denmark and the NHS, questions remain over whether in the longer-term the private sector, governed by competition and choice, will be focused on competing for cost or for quality (van Ginneken 2006; Knottnerus and ten Velden 2007). While yet to be implemented, the German government has also been looking at reforms designed to inject greater competition into its social insurance system. These reforms aim to extend insurance to the small percentage of people without coverage, and to improve coordination of care among providers (Lisac 2006).

Inadvertently, competitive practices have re-entered the New Zealand health system. As discussed above and in Chapter 2, competition and choice were integral to the neoliberal-influenced health system reforms of the early 1990s. Since then, the health system has been undergirded by social democratic ideals. The government's preference has been for devolved planning and funding through 21 local DHBs. These are contractually obligated to deliver on government policy within predetermined and restricted funding. Thus, at the local level, and required to prioritize and produce initiatives to save money, boards have reverted to the use of competitive markets and the private sector although there has been no move to stimulate patient choice. For example, several boards aiming for cost savings have closed their own laboratories and put laboratory testing up for tender. This has naturally expanded the role and size of the private sector.

CONCLUSION

This chapter overviewed the role of the private sector in health systems. This role varies across different systems and service issues and, as the chapter discussed, is contentious. This is because the private sector is frequently viewed as placing profits ahead of patients. Governments have also often looked to the private sector in the belief that it offers more efficient and better quality services while reducing demand on the public sector. The chapter, lastly, looked at renewed government interest, particularly in Britain, in emphasizing market concepts and private service delivery. This interest has placed the private sector firmly on the new health policy agenda.

Two issues make the recommitment to private sector ideals remarkable. First, is the fact that the earlier neoliberal era flirtations with markets and the private sector were largely unsuccessful and even damaging for affected health systems, including in Britain and New Zealand. For such reasons, they were shortlived. Second, is that the evidence supporting market notions and private sector involvement is weak. As the chapter noted, certain fields such as pharmaceuticals may be more suited to private dominance. When it comes to health services funding and organization the evidence mostly points away from private models. At best, private not-for-profit examples such as the fully integrated Kaiser system could have lessons for public health system improvement. At worst, it could be considered unfortunate that the broader US experience has been overlooked. Yet, in the British case the NHS is effectively being turned into a de-integrated system. As Hunter notes, this has occurred through a debate in which market advocates have had the stronger voice and ear of politicians (Hunter 2008). If history repeats itself, and if the 'market' fails to deliver, the result could be a difficult process of reversing structures designed for competition and choice. The same might be expected for other European countries pursuing market concepts. New Zealand's local pursuit of private sector mechanisms, in spite of a central government commitment to public services, could also be difficult to unravel.

A notable difference with the neoliberal era is the intent behind current market-oriented policies. The British case shows that aims have generally been to improve service standards and accessibility, and respond to the social democratic notion outlined in Chapter 1 that individuals should be as free as possible from state intervention and able to make choices that fit with their preferences. Aims have therefore also included expanding private provision. Whatever the intent, embracing the private sector or market mechanisms to pursue social democratic goals makes for complicated health systems and analysis. The next chapter discusses how, in theoretical terms, this complexity might be understood.

QUESTIONS FOR FURTHER DISCUSSION

1. What are some of the different ways that the private sector is involved in delivering health care?
2. What sorts of services should be privately provided and should there be limits on private sector involvement?
3. Will private sector ideals such as competition and choice improve public health systems?
4. Is the application of competition and choice driven by neoliberalism or social democracy, or some combination of the two; or are there other motivations?

8

CONCLUSION

The opening chapter of this book outlined a contextual framework for understanding health policy developments in many developed democratic countries today. The framework incorporated both theoretical and practical considerations. Theoretical considerations included the notion that there has been something of a transition in many countries from the influences of neoliberalism to those of social democracy. However, the remnants of neoliberal-inspired policies remain, and in several cases have continued to be promoted.

The combination of neoliberal and social democratic sentiments as a backdrop for policy offers an explanation for why governments might be interested in issues such as improving service access and reducing inequalities in health outcomes, but also in increasing accountability and control and promoting the role of the private sector and competition in health care systems. The combination also means that a range of organizational forms might be evident including traditional hierarchical bureaucracies, networks, partnership arrangements, and the use or creation of markets. The practical considerations that the framework included were around the implications of demographic change, increasing service demand but limited funding for this, the emergence of new diseases and health risks such as diabetes, obesity and SARS, and concerns about health system improvement and the quality and safety of health care.

The six core subject chapters in the book overviewed issues that are pivotal to health policy in many countries today. As noted in the introduction, these represent but a few of the possible topics that might be covered in a health policy book. However, as each of the respective chapters illustrated, they are 'big' issues that most developed world governments are grappling with, along with international agencies such as the OECD and the WHO. In this sense, the subject chapters represent essential components of a new health policy agenda.

This concluding chapter aims to:

- Highlight key themes and lessons from the policy issues covered in the core subject chapters
- Discuss the analytical framework set out in Chapter 1, particularly the intersection of neoliberalism and social democracy
- Consider the emerging organizational patterns discussed in Chapter 1 in the light of the material in the core chapters
- Suggest how the new health policy agenda might be subjected to further analysis.

SOME KEY THEMES

Several themes emerge from the material in the preceding chapters. This section highlights a selection.

The first theme is that links can be found between each of the core subject areas. As noted in Chapter 2, funding and organizational policies are increasingly oriented toward addressing the issues at the centre of subsequent chapters. Contemporary concerns include the desire for services to be better coordinated and patient centred but also designed to improve the quality of care delivered, and to reduce health inequalities and the burden of chronic disease. Quality improvement, as noted in Chapter 3, is in part contingent upon funding and organizational models that promote attention to care processes and service coordination. Chronic disease and inequality reduction are similarly dependent.

Policy makers are also pursuing ways to improve the efficiency or 'performance' of health systems and there has been interest in doing so by enhancing the role of provider competition and patient choice, especially in countries such as Britain and Denmark as discussed in Chapter 7. The notion of patient choice, of course, also chimes with concepts encapsulated by clinical governance. This embraces the idea that health professionals should be focused on improving patient care, while also involving patients as participants at all stages of the care process. Thus, where the neoliberal era as described in Chapter 1 saw models that may have simply been a means to an end (of increasing competition and choice per se), the period that followed has seen the emergence of a symbiotic relationship between how health care is funded and organized and a series of practical health system and service concerns.

A second theme is that there continues to be tensions among the approaches for tackling the issues in each of the subject chapters. Such tensions are illustrated in the example of quality improvement where, as noted in Chapter 3, policy makers may use a combination of both shame and blame and continuous quality improvement techniques as is the case in Britain. Similar tensions can be seen in the emergence of new professionalism, with professional bodies prompted into action by the impending threat of government regulation. Yet professionals remain wary of demands for patient involvement as touched on in Chapter 5. The lack of evidence that involvement policies improve patient care could well exacerbate professional concerns. Tensions are also evident in the application of ICT, the topic of Chapter 4. There are questions over failure rates of large ICT projects and therefore whether these are appropriate investments, or whether a series of smaller independent projects may produce better results. There are also tensions around the different uses of health care ICT systems. Management, for example, may have quite different perspectives from clinical staff.

Public health is another area prone to tensions, especially around the resourcing and locus of responsibility for health improvement. Britain's experience, discussed in Chapter 6, shows how Health Action Zones were undermined by inadequate funding and a shift in government policy away from tackling inequalities to individual responsibillity and targeting. Funding constraints mean that few intended links between New Zealand's District Health Boards and other health influencing sectors have been developed. At a global level, tensions are likely to increase around how to deal with issues relating to climate change, especially the impact on the developing world, and the inequalities among and within societies. Chapter 7 overviewed the ongoing tensions over the role of the private sector, particularly around whether it is more efficient than the public sector and capable, through competition and choice, of fulfilling goals of health system improvement.

A third theme is that there is a diversity of approaches to dealing with the core subject issues. As others have noted, this makes for complex comparative policy work (e.g. Scott 2001; Blank and Burau 2004; Gauld 2005a). Through brief illustrations, this book has looked at experiences from a limited range of countries. While these point to comparable approaches in some areas, there are considerable differences in others. Examples include the convergence in approaches to funding and organization in Britain and New Zealand in the neoliberal era, yet quite different tactics in the subsequent period where the British government has pursued private involvement and competition while New Zealand has tended to favour public sector services and collaboration. Britain has opted for a national strategy for quality improvement, while New Zealand has largely made this a local planning responsibility. Britain has been almost alone in creating new oversight bodies specifically intended to drive improvement of various aspects of NHS performance. The ways in which patients might be involved in service planning and delivery also differ. Britain has long experimented with patient forums, while New Zealand has created elected health boards and regulatory requirements that service governance bodies and planners routinely engage in public consultation. In the US, public involvement policies are notably absent, but some hospitals actively seek patient input into their work.

Private sector involvement is an area where comparisons are particularly difficult. In many countries, the private sector is the supplier of pharmaceuticals, albeit with government as a key purchaser, although, as discussed elsewhere, such purchasing arrangements differ from country to country (Callahan and Wasunna 2006: Chapter 5). When it comes to service funding and organization, variations are considerable. Private arrangements dominate the US health system, with little if any interaction between private and public organizations. Britain has opted for independent private treatment centres, funded by the NHS, while in the Netherlands the private sector provides the backbone of the social insurance system. In South Korea, public social insurance pays for a largely private service provision system. In Denmark, patients can choose private care where the public sector is unable to do so within a specified timeframe. In several countries, public funding is used to subsidize the services of private primary care medical practitioners whose fees would otherwise pose a considerable patient access barrier.

Following on from the above, a fourth theme is a lack of definitive answers in terms of how to deal with the subject chapter issues. The diversity in responses and inherent tensions within suggests that there is not necessarily any one best alternative to pursue when seeking to, for instance, improve quality or patient choice, or to better coordinate care or promote population health. Instead, policy directions are often influenced by local context including the extent to which policy makers emphasize issues and options and to which they are able to enact change. The British and New Zealand political systems permit wide-ranging and radical change, while policy makers in the US must work within a system designed to create obstacles. Pre-existing institutional arrangements provide an additional constraint. Due to tradition and 'path dependency' existing conditions are often impossible to eradicate and so, instead, policy is built upon arrangements already in place (Wilsford 1994). As outlined in Chapter 5, a prime example of this is the way in which the NHS public and patient involvement initiatives have followed a model first initiated in 1974. The main changes since have been around organization. Quality improvement in the US is another example of what may be a very gradual process of influencing existing and firmly-established organizations and practices. Similarly, the embeddedness of private financing arrangements in the US means that any reforms to its health system need to build on these foundations.

Fifth, as all the subject chapters imply, governments are inevitably becoming more involved in health care policy and systems. This is due to the growing complexity of health care provision, the changes in society that are creating pressures for policy makers as outlined in Chapter 1, and the very nature of the issues in the subject chapters. As Chapter 6 illustrated, there has been a gradual shift in thinking about public health. New public health philosophy, which many governments have adopted, requires proactive state involvement across a range of areas including housing, education and local government. So too does the widespread concern for inequality and for chronic diseases. Globalization and issues such as climate change have brought public health and environmental concerns to the fore, requiring government responses in both their own domestic arena as well as on the international stage. As Chapter 6 discussed, new thinking especially around transport and energy production is required. Globalization of communicable diseases such as SARS, and non-communicable diseases including diabetes and heart disease, is also demanding increasing government attention. Other issues propelling governments include the quality reports outlined in Chapter 3, evidence that ICT can improve various facets of health care delivery and system performance (Chapter 4), demands for improved professional governance (Chapter 5), and beliefs that the private sector may help improve system quality and efficiency (Chapter 7).

A sixth theme is that relationships between government, the private sector, health care professionals and patients are in a state of transition. The sovereignty of patients is being propelled by the emphasis on involvement initiatives, but also by developments in quality, ICT and the rekindling of market structures. In tandem, professionals are increasingly looking to patients and the public for legitimacy, particularly around service governance and configuration and professional standards. The British and other European country experiences suggest that there is potential for the private sector to be viewed as crucial to improvements in health services, meaning increasingly variegated health systems. Across all of the subjects canvassed in this book, government is playing a pivotal role. In Britain and New Zealand, central powers have been commanded to reform the health system. However, beyond structural reforms, these and other governments have increasingly moved into a 'stewardship' position (Saltman and Ferroussier-Davis 2000), forging strategic directions in areas such as quality, ICT and public health and attempting to influence the activities of service providers. Where possible, as in Britain and New Zealand, and with some variation, they have created national targets and goals, along with requirements that local level planners and providers work to deliver on these. In the US, stewardship has involved both federal and state governments facilitating initiatives such as extending health insurance.

A final theme, of course, is that several lessons for policy makers can be gleaned from the discussions in the core chapters. Many of these lessons are relevant to specific subjects. Quality improvement efforts, for example, could be counterproductive if the focus is wholly on shaming and blaming of those responsible for errors and substandard care, or if efforts lack leadership and coordination. ICT projects are likely to run into difficulty without careful organization and control throughout all developmental phases. Problems might also be expected where health professionals are not adequately consulted in the planning and implementation of new ICT systems. As Chapter 5 discussed, the implementation of clinical governance requires care so as to promote health professional support for such directions. Public and patient involvement initiatives, similarly, need to be carefully handled so that they do not unduly benefit only those who directly participate.

There are also lessons from the subject chapters as a whole. A key one, discussed elsewhere, is that policy-making is a 'messy' business (John 1998: 7). This is due to the history of developments in the policy area which, as noted above, will often provide the foundations on which new policies must inevitably be built. Policy is also messy because of the range of different and, as this book shows, often conflicting options for change available. Selected options often hinge on value judgements of decision makers which, in turn, will be grounded in theories (and/or evidence) about what kind of strategy may be the most effective (Howlett and Ramesh 1995). The role of the private sector, as discussed in Chapter 7, provides a pertinent example of this. Despite a lack of firm evidence that its strategy will be successful, Britain has opted to use the private sector to create competition among providers and choice for patients. Policies, of course, also need to be implemented which adds to the disorderliness (Hill and Hupe 2002). The implementation of funding and organizational changes in Britain and New Zealand overviewed in Chapter 2 are characteristic demonstrations of this. So too is the process of developing clinical governance discussed in Chapter 5. Any government, such as Britain's, that is in tandem pursuing each of the issues canvassed in the core subject chapters is faced with a picture of unparalleled complexity. Because of the messiness, it is difficult to find perfectly crafted and highly successful policies that can simply be emulated elsewhere without adaptation. In short, the lesson is probably that governments executing the new health policy agenda face a potentially bewildering array of policy development and implementation challenges.

NEOLIBERALISM, SOCIAL DEMOCRACY AND 'SOCIALIZED NEOLIBERALISM'

Chapter 1 outlined two philosophies – neoliberalism and social democracy – that have underpinned health policy in the 'reform' and 'post-reform' eras. This section looks at the extent to which the two philosophies have influenced policy in the areas covered in the core subject chapters and how, in theoretical terms, the intersection of these two philosophical positions might be explained.

As the discussions in each of the core chapters implied, developments in each of the areas under scrutiny have been influenced by a range of factors. Practical concerns could most certainly be seen as a crucial influence in several of the policy areas. The medical error studies outlined in Chapter 3 probably provide the most poignant example of this. The governance and accountability failures discussed in Chapter 5 and proof of the increasing burden of chronic disease are other illustrations. In other cases, the gradual availability of evidence and information on practical initiatives have been motivators for policy. ICT is a case in point with a mounting number of studies and service delivery experiences demonstrating that it can make a multifaceted contribution to health care systems. Such evidence presents an undeniable case that policy makers should become involved in promoting ICT development. Of course, evidence around issues such as climate change, or of the performance of organizations such as Kaiser Permanente, provides a similar motivation for policy.

Practical explanations may be less applicable to other subjects covered in the core chapters which is where theoretical explanations may prove their value. Several developments as described in each of the core chapters had clearly been influenced at least in part by the theories outlined in Chapter 1. Chapter 2 discussed how funding and organizational concerns are with accountability and managerial control as well as with facilitating responses to the issues in subsequent chapters. The chapter showed how governments, particularly in Britain and New Zealand, restructured their health systems in accordance with theoretical trends: initially under the influence of neoliberalism; and later propelled by social democratic thought. Chapter 2 also illustrated how both neoliberalism and social democracy had influenced present developed world health policy, especially in Britain. Other chapters also looked at the the influence of neoliberal and social democratic concepts. Both could be seen in the conjoining of shame and blame and CQI approaches to quality improvement. Both were evident in the managerial and service improvement aspects of ICT application. Both could be found in developments in clinical governance (demands for accountability combined with professional empowerment) and in approaches to public health improvement (target setting with financial inducements aimed at services intended to promote better health). A particularly strong influence of both neoliberalism and social democracy could be found in policies regarding the private sector (boosting availability of publicly-funded services via competitive market arrangements). As such, there is a case for confirming the combined influence of neoliberalism and social democracy on aspects of the new health policy agenda.

This raises the question of how, in theoretical terms, the seemingly incongruous combination of neoliberalism and social democracy might be explained. One possibility is that the directions of some governments and their approaches to health policy issues have been shaped by an emerging 'socialized neoliberalism' in which aspects of both neoliberalism and social democracy are drawn upon. The two philosophical positions have intersected via government which is traditionally social democratic and in pursuit of a policy agenda aimed at enhancing social policy, developing state capacity in this area and generally working to improve the lives and environments of citizens. Such a government would also hold fast to institutional arrangements developed and grounded in neoliberal principles, or apply neoliberal tools in pursuit of social democratic policy outcomes.

Tony Blair's British New Labour government was probably the classic exponent of socialized neoliberalism. The Blair government became known for its 'third way' approach to policy which was largely about the 'renewal' of social democracy in Britain. In this spirit, it forged a policy agenda aimed at democratizing government (Driver and Martell 2006). It espoused notions of an inclusive economy with the reduction of inequalities at the centre so that all people could be active participants. It sought to build an active civil society with improved public environments. It also pursued the idea of a partnership between citizens and government, with increased powers to deliver services devolved to local communities and service providers. The Blair government aimed to alleviate deprivation and poverty and sought to 'enable' people to live independently in the community (Taylor 2000).

In tandem, through its modernization programme, Blair's government sought improvements in public service efficiency and in transparency and openness. With the expanding reach of the state came demands for increased central government control and accountability for public money, paving the way for continuation of institutions and recommitment to policy tools designed around neoliberal principles. The Blair government became almost obsessive with oversight and, from the top-down, established a series of offices to drive new policy initiatives and applied performance targets to this. Value-for-money became a core concern, with associated requirements for proof that this was being delivered by public service providers (Geddes and Martin 2000).

If socialized neoliberalism provides an appropriate explanation, its utility may vary in two ways. First, at the level of the different policy areas overviewed in each of the individual chapters of this book. As discussed above, the theory may offer a better explanation for influences in funding and organization, and in private sector policy, than it does for consideration of public health issues and policy. This is not unusual as some policy areas will always be more conducive to theoretically-framed explanation.

The second way socialized neoliberalism's utility might vary is in its relevance to developments across different countries. In looking at Britain, New Zealand and the US, the primary points of comparison through this book, some notable contrasts could be found. Socialized neoliberalism may well offer a better framework for understanding developments in Britain and in a relatively consistent pattern across several of the subject areas covered in this book. Socialized neoliberalism may provide less of an explanation for developments in New Zealand and the US and may simply serve as a backdrop for thinking through the varying philosophical influences. As such, analysis of the impact of the practical issues outlined in Chapter 1 may also provide a useful point of reference.

It needs to be acknowledged that the combination of neoliberalism and social democracy that socialized neoliberalism brings together encompasses a range of influences and perspectives. In this way, it provides an organizing framework that incorporates 'polytheories' (a range of differing theories) which, as Oberlander implies, were required in his case for investigating the convoluted and evolving history of the US Medicare system (Oberlander 2003: 11). The extent to which a theory such as socialized neoliberalism can be applied to such a wide range of 'new health policy' issues across different developed world health systems and policies will always be open to debate and, naturally, demands further research. Of course, most theories generate only a partial explanation of events. Their primary value therefore is in offering a heuristic framework for exploring the dynamic and shifting influences in different policy areas, highlighting those in which theoretical influences are more prevalent.

EMERGING ORGANIZATIONAL MODELS

Chapter 1 listed four organizational forms for health care delivery. These were the traditional hierarchy, market-based models, networks, and partnership arrangements. Based on the discussions through the core chapters, this section considers the emerging modes of organization.

Each of the organizational forms appeared to be in existence around each of the subject areas. The funding and organization issues outlined in Chapter 2 illustrate this. Large hierarchical bureaucracies, such as NHS Trusts or New Zealand's District Health Boards, remain in each of the health systems discussed. However, in pursuit of the 'new health policy' issues outlined in Chapter 2 and in subsequent chapters, such organizations are increasingly involved in partnerships with other providers such as private primary care practitioners and independent service providers. They are contracting for services and so function in a market-like environment. In some cases, they are tendering for service contracts from funding bodies; in others, they are seeking service delivery from among competing providers. The presence of networks is also evident. An example is New Zealand's Primary Health Organizations. These contract for delivery of publicly-funded services in a benign but competitive atmosphere, and also network various primary care providers involved in delivering comprehensive services to diverse populations. Increasingly, communities are being included in these networks as new professionalism and clinical governance arrangements extend to involve the public in service planning and decision-making.

Quality is another area that features a collage of organizational arrangements. Large bureaucracies can be found, often where a national approach to a policy issue is required. Examples include Britain's various national organizations designed to drive quality improvement, or the US Agency for Healthcare Research and Quality. Of course, quality improvement strategies include reform of large bureaucratic hospital organizations. Quality also extends to involving patients in partnerships to improve care processes, integrating or building networks between public and private providers and hospital and primary care, as well as attempts to boost quality by resorting to market solutions of competing providers vying for patients.

The case of ICT shows how hierarchies can be pivotal to success, at least in terms of ensuring that policies and developments, across a network of inter-linked providers, are coordinated. ICT also illustrates how technology is increasingly driving networks and partnerships, but also capable of providing infrastructure for market-like scenarios. The NHS ICT programme is fundamental to enabling patients to check the quality and background of service providers, make choices among them and then book service appointments with preferred providers from either the public or private sectors.

Clinical governance, professionalism and public involvement arrangements also illustrate how national agencies as well as networks and community-driven partnerships can co-exist and form a part of the landscape. Again, the NHS provides examples with the Healthcare Commission and NICE helping to steer NHS professional standards and practices. Policies to involve the public and patients in health services planning have seen the emergence of a network of patient forums linked to NHS trusts. The new professionalism will also inherently require that practitioners work more closely together, as being propelled by evidence in the US, monitoring one another's standards of practice in loose network arrangements, but also that practitioners work in partnership with their patients.

Public health, as Chapter 6 outlined, is a field which by nature demands partnerships and network arrangements. Such arrangements sit at the core of the new public health agenda with its emphasis on building community and social determinants of health. However, all developed countries feature public health bureaucracies responsible for national disease monitoring and control. The organization of these agencies is nonetheless evolving as illustrated by the case of the US Centers for Disease Control which is partnering with state governments and communities around initiatives to reduce chronic disease. The application of market concepts also features in contemporary public health. Britain, New Zealand and other countries discussed in Chapter 6 are attaching targets to public health concerns and often binding service providers under contract to focus on these.

When it comes to the private sector market models naturally prevail with private providers, such as pharmaceutical and medical device companies developing products and services that will be lucrative. However, other organizational forms may also be found such as public-private partnerships and arrangements (that could be deemed either natural market practices or loose networks) where public services work contiguously with private services. Such a case can be found in the creation of Britain's independent sector treatment centres where, as discussed in Chapter 7, NHS staff are working on secondment to private service providers. Other health systems, such as New Zealand, feature similar arrangements, with public hospital specialists maintaining parallel private practices. The private sector is also notable for the interface with the public sector where large bureaucracies, such as a health ministry or social insurance agency, may contract with or be involved in scrutinizing the standards and activities of private providers.

Perhaps the clearest organizational pattern emerging from the subjects covered in this book is one of multiplicity; of differing models of organization around each issue which depend on the preferences of politicians (who may prefer competitive market-based, or public sector and collaborative solutions), service planners and managers seeking optimal organizational solutions, and the traditions within countries. This scenario, of course, is in keeping with the suggestion in Chapter 1 that all organizational forms are likely in contemporary health systems.

CONCLUSION: A NEW HEALTH POLICY
RESEARCH AGENDA

This book has implied that there is a new health policy agenda. This agenda constitutes a series of policy issues of concern to most developed world governments and also to international agencies. Each of the core subject chapters provided a background to the issue under study that noted its importance. This concluding chapter has highlighted the fact that the issues are interrelated.

As discussed through this book, each of the core subject issues may be seen as being driven by a combination of factors, some more so than others. This combination, at least in the countries covered in the book, includes the influences of neoliberalism and social democracy, in addition to practical imperatives. Despite a view that ICT, for example, may represent attempts to subsume health care professionals under a managerial control system, or propel clinicians to more closely engage with increasingly Internet-educated patients, there is simple evidence that ICT improves health care quality (Chaudry et al. 2006). As noted previously in this chapter, this makes for complex analysis but demonstrates how both theoretical and practical concerns need to be considered. Evidence can also be cited as a rationale for quality improvement or for enhancing the conditions that people live in, despite the fact that both could be seen as being motivated by theoretical concerns or the demands of advocacy groups.

If there is a new health policy agenda, as outlined in this book, it needs to be subjected to additional analysis. This book is a start and leaves many questions unanswered. There is a demand for additional research into how policy makers incorporate both neoliberal and social democratic aspirations into their policies and whether such a combination is appropriate. More comparative country work would be useful in order to examine the robustness and dynamics of the topics on new health policy agenda. It may be beneficial to consider whether other analytical frameworks provide a better lens through which to understand contemporary health policy developments both within countries and comparatively. It might be useful, for instance, to look at the issues covered in this book via Esping-Andersen's 'world's of welfare capitalism' framework (Esping-Andersen 1990), or to apply Gilbert's argument that the state's role has shifted from being a provider to an 'enabler' of services (Gilbert 2002). The widely used approach of analysing how actors at different levels of health systems – regulators, funders and providers – deal with each of the issues could also be applied (Mossialos et al. 2002; Holliday and Wilding 2003; Gauld 2005a). Analysis might additionally consider the extent to which responses to the issues are influenced by North American political values. As Moran argued of the neoliberal era, markets were increasingly being used for government resource allocation, and the power of the medical profession eroded by progressively innovative purchasers (Moran 1994). It could be valuable to consider whether this argument has been sustained and even rejuvenated in the subsequent era. Finally, the influence and utility of the concept of socialized neoliberalism could be studied through a range of additional policy topics.

References

Abelson, J., J. Eyles, C.B. McLeod, P. Collins, C. McMullan, and P-G. Forest (2003) Does deliberation make a difference? Results from a citizens panel study of health goals priority setting, *Health Policy*, 66: 95–106.

ABIM Foundation, ACP-ASIM Foundation and Eurpoean Federation of Internal Medicine (2002) Medical professionalism in the new millennium: a physician charter, *Annals of Internal Medicine*, 136(3): 243–6.

Abraham, T. (2005) *Twenty-first Century Plague: The Story of SARS*. Baltimore, CA: Johns Hopkins University Press.

Acheson, D. (1998) *Independent Inquiry into Inequalities in Health*. London: Stationery Office.

Advisory Council on Health Infostructure (1999) *Canada Health Infoway: Paths to Better Health*. Ottowa: Advisory Council on Health Infostructure.

Ahern, M., Kovats, R.S., Wilkinson, P., Few, R. and Matthies, F. (2005) Global health impacts of floods: epidemiologic evidence, *Epidemiologic Reviews*, 27(1): 36–46.

Allin, S., Mossialos, E., McKee, M. and Holland, W. (2004) *Making Decisions on Public Health: A Review of Eight Countries*. Brussels: European Observatory on Health Systems and Policy.

Altenstetter, C. and Warner Bjorkman, J. (eds) (1997) *Health Policy Reform, National Variations and Globalization*. Houndmills: Macmillan.

Anderson, G.F., Frogner, B.K., Johns, R.A. and Reinhardt, U.E. (2006) Health care spending and use of information technology in OECD countries, *Health Affairs*, 25(3): 819–31.

Anderson, J.G., Rainey, M.R. and Eysenbach, G. (2003) The impact of cyberhealthcare on the physician-patient relationship, *Journal of Medical Systems*, 27(1): 67–84.

Anton, S., McKee, L., Harrison, S. and Farrar, S. (2007) Involving the public in NHS service planning, *Journal of Health Organization and Management,* 21 (4/5): 470–83.

Arah, O.A., Westert, G.P., Hurst, J. and Klazinga, N.S. (2006) A conceptual framework for the OECD health care quality indicators project, *International Journal for Quality in Health Care*, 18(1): 5–13.

Arnstein, S. (1969) A ladder of participation, *Journal of the American Institute of Planners*, July: 216–23.

Asher, M.G. and Nandy, A. (2006) Health financing in Singapore: a case for systemic reforms, *International Social Security Journal*, 59(1): 75–92.

Ashton, J. and Seymour, H. (1988) *The New Public Health*. Milton Keynes: Open University Press.

Asthana, S. and Halliday, J. (2006) *What Works in Tackling Health Inequalities? Pathways, Policies and Practice Through the Life-course*. Bristol: The Policy Press.

Ayanian, J.Z., Weissman, J.S., Schneider, E.C., Ginsberg, J.A. and Zaslavsky, A.M. (2000) Unmet health needs of uninsured adults in the United States, *Journal of the American Medical Association*, 284: 2061–9.

Baker, A. (2007) Patient involvement in a professional body: reflections and commentary, *Journal of Health Organization and Management*, 21(4/5): 460–9.

Bandaranayake, D. (1994) Public health and the reforms: the New Zealand experience, *Health Policy*, 29(1–2): 127–41.

Barr, D.A. (2007) A research protocol to evaluate the effectiveness of public-private partnerships as a means to improve health and welfare systems worldwide, *American Journal of Public Health*, 97(1): 19–25.

Barr, M.D. (2005) Singapore, in R. Gauld (ed.) *Comparative Health Policy in the Asia-Pacific*. Maidenhead: Open University Press.

Bate, P. and Robert, G. (2006) Experience-based design: from redesigning the system around the patient to co-designing services with the patient, *Quality and Safety in Health Care*, 15: 307–10.

Bauer, S., Percevic, R., Okon, E., Meermann, R. and Kordy, H. (2003) Use of text messaging in the aftercare of patients with bulimia nervosa, *European Eating Disorders Review*, 11(3): 279–90.

Bauld, L. and K. Judge, eds. 2002. *Learning from Health Action Zones*. Chichester: Aeneas Press.

Baum, F. (2002) *The New Public Health,* 2nd edn. Melbourne: Oxford University Press.

Baum, F. (2008) *The New Public Health,* 3rd edn. Melbourne: Oxford University Press.

Beaglehole, R. (ed.) (2003) *Global Public Health: A New Era.* Oxford: Oxford University Press.

Beaglehole, R. and Bonita, R. (1997) *Public Health at the Crossroads: Achievements and Prospects.* Cambridge: Cambridge University Press.

Beaglehole, R. and Yach, D. (2003) Globalisation and the prevention and control of non-communicable disease: the neglected chronic diseases of adults, *The Lancet,* 362: 903–8.

Benson, L.A., Boyd, A. and Walshe, K. (2006) Learning from regulatory interventions in healthcare: the commission for health improvement and its clinical governance review process, *Clinical Governance: An International Journal,* 11(3): 213–24.

Berg, M. (2004) *Health Information Management: Integrating Information Technology in Health Care Work.* London: Routledge.

Berwick, D. (2002) A user's manual for the IOM's 'Quality Chasm' Report, *Health Affairs,* 21(3): 80–90.

Bevan, G. and Hood, C. (2006) Have targets improved performance in the English NHS? *British Medical Journal,* 332: 419–22.

Bird, S.M., Cox, D., Farewell, Goldstein, H., Hold, T. and Smith, P.C, (2005) Performance indicators: good, bad, and ugly, *Journal of the Royal Statistical Society,* 168: 1–27.

Blakely, T., Tobias, M., Atkinson, J., Yeh, L-C. and Huang, K. (2007) *Tracking Disparity: Trends in Ethnic and Socioeconomic Inequalities in Mortality, 1981–2004.* Wellington: Ministry of Health.

Blakely, T., Tobias, M., Robson, B., Ajwani, S., Bonne, M. and Woodward, A. (2005) Widening ethnic mortality disparities in New Zealand 1981–99, *Social Science & Medicine* 61(10): 2233–51.

Blank, R.H. and Burau, V. (2004) *Comparative Health Policy.* Houndmills: Palgrave Macmillan.

Blendon, R.J., Brodie, M., Benson, J.M., Altman, D.E., Levitt, L., Hoff, T. and Hugick, L. (1998) Understanding the managed care backlash, *Health Affairs* 17(4): 80–94.

Blumenthal, D. and Glaser, J. (2007) Information technology comes to medicine, *New England Journal of Medicine,* 356(24): 2527–34.

Bodenheimer, T. (2008) Coordinating care: a perilous journey through the health system, *New England Journal of Medicine,* 358(10): 1064–71.

Bogdanor, V. (ed.) (2005) *Joined-Up Government*. Oxford: The British Academy and Oxford University Press.

Boston, J., Dalziel, P. and St John, S. (eds) (1999) *Redesigning the Welfare State in New Zealand: Problems, Policies, Prospects*. Auckland: Oxford University Press.

Brennan, T.A., Leape, L., Laird, N.M., et al. (1991) Incidence of adverse events and negligence in hospitalized patients: results of the Harvard medical practice study, *New England Journal of Medicine*, 324(6): 370–6.

Bristol Royal Infirmary Inquiry (2001) *Learning from Bristol: The Report of the Public Inquiry into Children's Heart Surgery at the Bristol Royal Infirmary 1984–1995*. London: Stationery Office.

Bruce, D.A. (2007) Regulation of doctors, *British Medical Journal*, 334: 346–437.

Buse, K. and Harmer, A. (2007) Seven habits of highly effective global public-private health partnerships: practice and potential, *Social Science & Medicine*, 64: 259–71.

Bush, G.W. (2004) *Transforming Health Care: The President's Health Information Technology Plan*. Washington DC: The White House.

Callahan, D. and Wasunna, A. (2006) *Medicine and the Market: Equity v. Choice*. Baltimore, CA: Johns Hopkins University Press.

Cameron, D. and Jones, I.G. (1983) John Snow, the Broad Street pump and modern epidemiology, *International Journal of Epidemiology*, 12(4): 393–6.

Campbell, S., Reeves, D., Kontopantelis, E., Middleton, E., Sibbald, B. and Roland, M. (2007) Quality of primary care in England with the introduction of pay for performance, *New England Journal of Medicine* 357(2): 181–90.

Carter, N., Klein, R. and Day, P. (1995) *How Organisations Measure Success: The Use of Performance Indicators in Government*. London: Routledge.

Cartwright, S. (1988) *The Report of the Cervical Cancer Inquiry*. Auckland: Government Printing Office.

Casilino, L., Gillies, R.R., Shortell, S.M. et al. (2003) External incentives, information technology, and organized processes to improve health care quality for patients with chronic diseases, *Journal of the American Medical Association*, 289 (4): 434–41.

Center for Evaluative Clinical Sciences (1998) *The Dartmouth Atlas of Health Care 1998*. Chicago: American Hospital Publishing.

Centers for Disease Control (2008) *Obesity and Overweight: State-Based Programs*. Atlanta: Centers for Disease Control.

Chadwick, A. and May, C. (2003) Interaction between states and citizens in the age of the internet: 'E-government' in the United States, Britain and the European Union, *Governance* 16(2): 271–300.

Chaudry, B., Wang, J., Wu, S. et al. (2006) Systematic review: impact of health information technology on quality, efficiency, and costs of medical care, *Annals of Internal Medicine*, 144: 742–52.

Chisholm, A., Redding, D., Cross, P. and Coulter, A. (2007) *Patient and Public Involvement in PCT Commissioning: A Survey of Primary Care Trusts.* Oxford: Picker Institute Europe.

Cohen, A.B., Restuccia, J.D., Shwartz, M., et al. (2008) A survey of hospital quality improvement activities, *Medical Care Research and Review*, 65(5): 571–95.

Cohen, D. (2008) English Trusts will be allowed to advertise their services, *British Medical Journal*, 336(7676): 685.

Commission on Social Determinants of Health (2007) *A Conceptual Framework for Action on the Social Determinants of Health. Discussion paper for the Commission on Social Determinants of Health*, April. Geneva: World Health Organization.

Commission on Social Determinants of Health (2008) *Closing the Gap in a Generation: Health Equity Through Action on the Social Determinants of Health.* Geneva: World Health Organization.

Committee for Economic Development (2007) *Quality, Affordable Health Care for All: Moving Beyond the Employer-Based Health-Insurance System.* Washington, DC: Committee for Economic Development.

Commonwealth Fund (2006) *Framework for a High Performance Health System for the United States.* New York: Commonwealth Fund.

Commonwealth Fund Commission on a High Performance Health System (2006) *Why Not the Best? Results from a National Scorecard on US Health System Performance.* New York: Commonwealth Fund.

Commonwealth Fund Commission on a High Performance Health System (2008) *Why Not the Best? Results from the National Scorecard on US Health System Performance.* New York: The Commonwealth Fund.

Cook, R.F., Billings, D.W., Hersch, R.K., Back, A.S. and Hendrickson, A. (2007) A field test of a web-based workplace health promotion program to improve dietary practices, reduce stress, and increase physical activity: randomized controlled trial, *Journal of Medical Internet Research*, 9: e17.

Coulter, A. (2002) After Bristol: putting patients at the centre, *Quality and Safety in Health Care*, 11: 186–8.

Crawford, M.J., Rutter, D., Manley, C., et al. (2002) Systematic review of involving patients in the planning and development of health care, *British Medical Journal*, 325: 1263–7.

Creech, W. (1999) *The Government's Medium-term Strategy for Health and Disability Support Services 1999*. Wellington: Ministry of Health.

Crosson, F. (2003) Kaiser permanente: a propensity for partnership, *British Medical Journal*, 326: 654.

Dalcher, D. and Genus, A. (2003) Avoiding IS/IT implementation failure, *Technology Analysis and Strategic Management*, 15(4): 403–7.

Davis, K., Schoen, C., Schoenbaum, S.C., et al. (2007) *Mirror, Mirror on the Wall: An International Update on the Comparative Performance of American Health Care*. New York: The Commonwealth Fund.

Davis, P. (2004) Tough but fair? The active management of the New Zealand drug benefits scheme by an independent crown agency, *Australian Health Review*, 28(2): 171–81.

Davis, P., Lay-Yee, R., Briant, R., et al. (2002) Adverse events in New Zealand Public hospitals: occurrence and impact, *New Zealand Medical Journal*, 115(1167).

DeAngelis, C. (2006) The influence of money on medical science, *Journal of the American Medical Association*, 296: 996–8.

Deming, W.E. (1986) *Out of the Crisis*. Boston: MIT Press.

Department of Health (1998) *A First Class Service: Quality in the New NHS*. London: Department of Health.

Department of Health (2000a) *An Organisation with a Memory. Report of an Expert Group on Learning from Adverse Events in the NHS*. London: Department of Health.

Department of Health (2001a) *Building a Safer NHS for Patients: Implementing an Organisation with a Memory*. London: Department of Health.

Department of Health (2001b) *Building the Information Core: Implementing the NHS Plan*. London: Department of Health.

Department of Health (2007) *Health Profile of England 2007*. London: Department of Health.

Department of Health (2008a) *Healthy Weight, Healthy Lives: A Cross Government Strategy for England*. London: HMSO.

Department of Health (2008b) *High Quality Care for All: NHS Next Stage Review FInal Report*. London: Department of Health.

Department of Health (1997) *The New NHS: Modern, Dependable.* London: Stationery Office.

Department of Health (2000b) *The NHS Plan: A Plan for Investment, A Plan for Reform.* London: The Stationery Office.

Department of Health (1989) *Working for Patients.* London: HMSO.

DesRoches, C.M., Campbell, E.G., Rao, S.R., et al. (2008) Electronic health records in ambulatory care: a national survey of physicians, *New England Journal of Medicine*, 358(28).

Devereaux, P.J., Heels-Ansdell, D., Lacchetti, C., et al. (2004) Payments for care at private for-profit and private not-for-profit hospitals: a systematic review and meta-analysis, *Canadian Medical Association Journal*, 170(12): 1817–24.

Devereaux, P.J., Schunemann, H.J., Ravindran, N., et al. (2002) Comparison of mortality between private for-profit and private not-for-profit hemodialysis centers: a systematic review and meta-analysis, *Journal of the American Medical Association*, 288(19): 2449–57.

Devlin, N., Maynard, A. and Mays, N. (2001) New Zealand's new health sector reforms: back to the future? *British Medical Journal*, 322(7295): 1171–4.

Dickerson, S., Reinhart, A.M., Feeley, T.H., Bidani, R., Garg, V. and Hershey, C.O. (2004) Patient Internet use for health information at three urban primary care clinics, *Journal of the American Health Informatics Association*, 11(6): 499–504.

District Health Boards New Zealand (2005) *PHO Performance Management Programme.* Wellington: District Health Boards New Zealand.

Donaldson, L. (2006) *Good Doctors, Safer Patients: Proposals to Strengthen the System to Assure and Improve the Performance of Doctors and to Protect the Safety of Patients.* London: Department of Health.

Driver, S. and Martell, L. (2006) *New Labour.* Cambridge: Polity Press.

Duckett, S. (2005) Australia, in R. Gauld (ed.) *Comparative Health Policy in the Asia-Pacific.* Maidenhead: Open University Press.

Dudley, R.A. and Luft, H.S. (2001) Managed care in transition, *New England Journal of Medicine*, 344(14): 1087–92.

Ellis, C.J. and White, H. (2006) Pharmac and the statin debate, *New Zealand Medical Journal*, 119 (1236).

Enthoven, A. (1985) *Reflection on the Management of the National Health Service.* London: Nuffield Provincial Hospitals Trust.

Enthoven, A. and van de Ven, W. (2007) Going Dutch: managed-competition health insurance in the Netherlands, *New England Journal of Medicine*, 357(24): 2421–3.

Epstein, A.M. (2006) Paying for performance in the United States and abroad, *New England Journal of Medicine*, 355: 406–8.

Esping-Andersen, G. (1990) *The Three Worlds of Welfare Capitalism*. Cambridge: Polity Press.

Exworthy, M., Berney, L. and Powell, M. (2002) How great expectations in Westminster may be dashed locally: the local implementation of national policy on health inequalities, *Policy and Politics*, 30(1): 79–96.

Eysenbach, G. and Kohler, C. (2002) How do consumers search for and appraise health information on the World Wide Web? Qualitative study using focus groups, usability tests, and in-depth interviews, *British Medical Journal*, 324: 572–7.

Eysenbach, G., Powell, J., Kuss, O. and Sa, E.R. (2002) Empirical studies assessing the quality of health information for consumers on the World Wide Web: a systematic review, *Journal of the American Medical Association*, 287: 2691–700.

Feachem, R., Sekhri, N. and White, K. (2002) Getting more for their dollar: a comparison of the NHS with California's Kaiser Permanente, *British Medical Journal*, 324: 135–43.

Ferris, J.D. (2005) Independent sector treatment centres (ISTCs): Early experience from an opthalmology service, *Eye*, 19: 1090–8.

Fidler, D.P. (2004) *SARS, Governance and the Globalization of Disease*. Houndmills: Palgrave Macmillan.

Figueras, J., Saltman, R.B., Busse, R. and Dubois, H.F.W. (2004) Patterns and performance in social health insurance systems, in R. B. Saltman, R. Busse and J. Figueras (eds) *Social Health Insurance Systems in Western Europe*. Maidenhead: Open University Press.

Fiscella, K., Franks, P., Gold, M.R. and Clancy, C.M. (2000) Inequality in quality: addressing socioeconomic, racial, and ethnic disparities in health care, *Journal of the American Medical Association*, 283(19): 2579–84.

Florin, D. and Dixon, J. (2004) Public involvement in health care, *British Medical Journal* 328: 159–61.

Flynn, R. (1992) *Structures of Control in Health Management*. London: Routledge.

Freeman, T. and Walshe, K. (2004) Achieving progress through clinical governance? A national study of health care managers' perceptions in the NHS in England, *Quality and Safety in Health Care*, 13: 335–43.

Fudge, N., Wolfe, C.D.A. and McKevitt, C. (2008) Assessing the promise of user involvement in health service development: ethnographic study, *British Medical Journal*, 336: 313–17.

Furstenbuerg, T., Rochell, T. Roeder, N. and Breithardt, G. (2007) Ambulatory and hospital care in the Federal Republic of Germany, *American Heart Hospital Journal*, 5(1): 22–6.

Gamble, V.N. and Stone, D. (2006) US policy on health inequities: the interplay of politics and research, *Journal of Health Politics, Policy and Law*, 31(1): 93–126.

Gauld, R. (2001) *Revolving Doors: New Zealand's Health Reforms.* Wellington: Institute of Policy Studies and Health Services Research Centre.

Gauld, R. (ed.) (2003) *Continuity amid Chaos: Health Care Management and Delivery in New Zealand.* Dunedin: University of Otago Press.

Gauld, R. (2004) One step forward, one step back? Restructuring, evolving policy and information technology and management in the New Zealand health sector, *Government Information Quarterly*, 21(2): 125–42.

Gauld, R. (ed.) (2005a) *Comparative Health Policy in the Asia-Pacific.* Maidenhead: Open University Press.

Gauld, R. (2005b) Delivering democracy? An analysis of New Zealand's district health board elections, 2001 and 2004, *Australian Health Review*, 29 (3): 245–352.

Gauld, R. (2005c) Exposing the cracks: severe acute respiratory syndrome and the Hong Kong health system, *Journal of Health Organization and Management*, 19(2): 106–19.

Gauld, R. (2005d) New Zealand, in R. Gauld (ed.) *Comparative Health Policy in the Asia-Pacific.* Maidenhead: Open University Press.

Gauld, R. (2007) Public sector information system project failures: lessons from a New Zealand hospital organization, *Government Information Quarterly* 24(1): 102–14.

Gauld, R. (2008a) Singapore's health system, in C. Aspalter, U. Yasuo and R. Gauld (eds) *Health Care Systems in Europe and Asia.* Taipei: Casa Verde.

Gauld, R. (2008b) The unintended consequences of New Zealand's primary care reforms, *Journal of Health Politics, Policy and Law*, 33(1): 93–117.

Gauld, R. and Goldfinch, S. (2006) *Dangerous Enthusiasms: E-Government, Computer Failure and Information System Development.* Dunedin: Otago University Press.

Gauld, R., Ikegami, N., Barr, M.D. et al. (2006) Advanced Asia's health systems in comparison, *Health* Policy, 79: 325–36.

Gauld, R. and Mays, N. (2006) Reforming primary care: are New Zealand's new primary health organisations fit for purpose? *British Medical Journal*, 333: 1216–18.

Geddes, M. and Martin, S. (2000) The policy and politics of best value: currents, crosscurrents and undercurrents in the new regime, *Policy and Politics*, 28 (3): 379–95.

General Medical Council (1995) *Good Medical Practice*. London: General Medical Council.

Gerth, H.H. and Mills, C.W. (eds) (1948) *From Max Weber: Essays in Sociology*. London: Routledge and Kegan Paul.

Gibbs, A., Fraser, D. and Scott, J. (1988) *Unshackling the Hospitals: Report of the Hospital and Related Services Taskforce*. Wellington: Hospital and Related Services Taskforce.

Giddens, A. (1998) *The Third Way: The Renewal of Social Democracy*. Cambridge: Polity Press.

Gilbert, N. (2002) *Transformation of the Welfare State: The Silent Surrender of Public Responsibility*. New York: Oxford University Press.

Glennester, H., Matsaganis, M., Owens, P. and Hancock, S. (1993) GP fundholding: wild card or hidden hand? In R. Robinson and J. Le Grand (eds) *Evaluating the NHS Reforms*. London: King's Fund Institute.

Gold, S.K.T., Abelson, J. and Charles, C.A. (2005) From rhetoric to reality: including patient voices in supportive cancer care planning, *Health Expectations* 8: 195–209.

Goldman, J. and Hudson, Z. (2000) Virtually exposed: privacy and e-health, *Health Affairs*, 19 (6): 140–9.

Gottlieb, S. (2004) US doctors want to be paid for email communication with patients, *British Medical Journal*, 328: 1155.

Gray, J.D. and Donaldson, L.J. (1996) Improving the quality of health care through contracting: a study of health authority practice, *Quality in Health Care*, 5: 201–5.

Griffiths, S. and Hunter, D.(2007) Introduction, in S. Griffiths and D. Hunter (eds) *New Perspectives in Public Health, 2nd edition*. Oxford: Radcliffe Publishing.

Haines, A., Kovats, R.S., Campbell-Lendrum, D. and Corvalan, C. (2006) Climate change and human health: impacts, vulnerability, and mitigation, *The Lancet*, 367: 2101–9.

Hales, S., de Wet, N., Macdonald, J. and Woodward, A. (2002) Potential effect of population and climate changes on global distribution of Dengue Fever: an empirical model, *The Lancet*, 360: 830–4.

Halligan, A. and Donaldson, L. (2001) Implementing clinical governance: turning vision into reality, *British Medical Journal*, 322: 1413–17.

Ham, C., (ed.) (1997) *Health Care Reform: Learning from International Experience*. Buckingham: Open University Press.

Ham, C. (2005) From targets to standards: but not just yet, *British Medical Journal*. 330: 106–7.

Ham, C. (2008) Competition and integration in the English National Health Service, *British Medical Journal*, 336: 805–7.

Ham, C., and Robert, G. (eds) (2003) *Reasonable Rationing: International Experience of Priority Setting in Health Care*. Buckingham: Open University Press.

Ham, C., York, N., Sutch, S. and Shaw, R. (2003) Hospital bed utilisation in the NHS, Kaiser Permanente, and the US Medicare Programme: analysis of routine data, *British Medical Journal*, 327: 1257–61.

Harrison, S., Milewa, T. and G. Dowswell (2002) Public and user 'involvement' in the National Health Service, *Health and Social Care in the Community*, 10(2): 1–4.

Hasnain-Wynia, R., Baker, D.W., Nerenz, D., et al. (2007) Disparities in health care are driven by where minority patients seek care, *Archives of Internal Medicine*, 167: 1233–9.

Hassenteufel, P. and Palier, B. (2007) Towards neo-Bismarckian health care states? Comparing health insurance reforms in Bismarckian welfare systems, *Social Policy and Administration*, 41(6): 574–96.

Hausman, D.M., Asada, Y. and Hedemann, T. (2002) Health inequalities and why they matter, *Health Care Analysis*, 10: 177–91.

Health Information Strategy Steering Committee (2005) *Health Information Strategy for New Zealand*. Wellington: Ministry of Health.

Heath, I., Hippisley-Cox, J. and Smeeth, L. (2007) Measuring performance and missing the point? *British Medical Journal*, 335: 1075–6.

Heeks, R. (2006) *Implementing and Managing E-Government: An International Text*. London: Sage Publications.

Held, D., and McGrew, A. (eds) (2000) *The Global Transformations Reader: An Introduction to the Globalization Debate*. Cambridge: Policy Press.

Herxheimer, A., McPherson, A., Miller, R., et al. (2000) A database of patients' experiences (DIPEx): new ways of sharing experience and information using a multimethod approach, *The Lancet*, 355: 1540–3.

Hill, A., Griffiths, S. and Gillam, S. (2007) *Public Health and Primary Care: Partners in Population Health*. Oxford: Oxford University Press.

Hill, M. and Hupe, P. (2002) *Implementing Public Policy*. London: Sage Publications.

Hillestad, R., Bigelow, J. and Bower, A. (2005) Can electronic medical record systems transform health care? Potential benefits, savings and costs, *Health Affairs*, 24(5): 1103–17.

Himmelstein, D., Warren, E. Thorne, D., et al. (2005) Illness and injury as contributors to bankruptcy, *Health Affairs*, web exclusive: w5-63-w5-73.

Himmelstein, D. and Woolhandler, S. (2001) *Bleeding the Patient: The Consequences of Corporate Health Care*. Monroe: Common Courage Press.

Hofmarcher, M.M., Oxley, H. and Rusticelli, E. (2007) *Improved Health System Performance Through Better Care Coordination. OECD Health Working Paper No. 30*. Paris: OECD.

Hogan, H., Basnett, I. and McKee, M. (2007) Consultants' attitudes to clinical governance: barriers and incentives to engagement, *Public Health*, 121: 614–22.

Hogg, C.N.L. (2007) Patient and public involvement: what next for the NHS? *Health Expectations*, 10: 129–38.

Holliday, I. and Wilding, P. (eds) (2003) *Welfare Capitalism in East Asia: Social Policy in the Tiger Economies*. Houndmills: Palgrave Macmillan.

Horton, R. (2001) The real lessons from Harold Frederick Shipman, *The Lancet* 357: 82–3.

Horton, R. (2005) The neglected epidemic of chronic disease, *The Lancet*, 366: 1514.

Houston, T.K., Sands, D.Z., Jenckes, M.W., et al. (2004) Experiences of patients who were early adopters of electronic communication with their physician: satisfaction, benefits, and concerns, *American Journal of Managed Care*, 10(9): 601–8.

Hovenga, E. and Lloyd, S. (2002) Working with information, in M. Harris (ed.) *Managing Health Services: Concepts and Practice*. Eastgardens, NSW : Maclennan and Petty.

Howlett, M. and Ramesh, M. (1995) *Studying Public Policy: Policy Cycles and Policy Subsystems*. Toronto: Oxford University Press.

Hummel, R.P. (1987) *The Bureaucratic Experience*. New York: St Martin's Press.

Hunter, D.J. (1994) From tribalism to corporatism: the managerial challenge to medical dominance, in J. Gabe, D. Kelleher and G. Williams (eds) *Challenging Medicine*. London: Routledge.

Hunter, D.J. (2008) *The Health Debate*. Bristol: The Policy Press.

Hussey, P., Anderson, G.F., Osborn, R., et al. (2004) How does the quality of care compare in five countries? *Health Affairs*, 23(3): 89–99.

Ikegami, N. (2005) Japan, in R. Gauld (ed.) *Comparative Health Policy in the Asia-Pacific*. Maidenhead: Open University Press.

Institute of Medicine (2001) *Crossing the Quality Chasm: A New Health System for the Twenty-First Century*. Washington: National Academy Press.

Institute of Medicine (2000) *To Err is Human: Building a Safer Health System*. Washington, DC: National Academy Press.

Institute of Medicine (2003) *Unequal Treatment: Confronting Racial and Ethnic Disparities in Health Care*. Washington, DC: National Academy Press.

Intergovernmental Panel on Climate Change (2001) *Climate Change 2001: Impacts, Adaptation and Vulnerability. Contribution of Working Group 1 to the Third Assessment Report of the Intergovernmental Panel on Climate Change*. Cambridge: Cambridge University Press.

Irvine, D. (2005) GMC and the future of revalidation: patients, professionalism and revalidation, *British Medical Journal*, 330: 1265–8.

Irvine, D. (1999) The performance of doctors: the new professionalism. *The Lancet*, 353: 1174–7.

Jacobson, M.Z., Colella, W.G. and Golden, D.M. (2005) Cleaning the air and improving health with hydrogen fuel-cell vehicles, *Science*, 308: 1901–5.

Jain, M., Miller, L., Belt, D., King, D. and Berwick, D. (2006) Decline in ICU adverse events, nosocomial infections and cost through a quality improvement initiative focusing on teamwork and culture change, *Quality and Safety in Health Care,* 15: 235–9.

James, J., Thomas, P. and Kerr, D. (2007) Preventing childhood obesity: two year follow-up results from the Christchurch obesity prevention programmes in schools (CHOPPS), *British Medical Journal*, 335: 762–4.

Jamtvedt, G., Young, J.M., Kristoffersen, D.T., O'Brien, M.A. and Oxman, A.D. (2006) Does telling people what they have been doing change what they do? A systematic review of the effects of audit and feedback, *Quality and Safety in Health Care*, 15: 433–6.

Jha, A.K., Ferris, T.G., Donelan, K., et al. (2006) How common are electronic health records in the United States? A summary of the evidence, *Health Affairs*, 25: w496–w507.

Jha, A.K., Orav, E.J., Li, Z. and Epstein, A.M. (2007) The inverse relationship between mortality rates and performance in the hospital quality alliance measures, *Health Affairs*, 26(4): 1104–10.

John, P. (1998) *Analysing Public Policy*. London: Continuum.

Jonas, S., Goldsteen, R. and Goldsteen, K. (2007) *An Introduction to the U.S. Health Care System*. New York: Springer Publishing Company.

Jones, I.R. (2003) Health professions, in G. Scambler (ed.) *Sociology as Applied to Medicine, 5th edn*. London: Elsevier.

Jost, T. (ed.) (2004) *Health Care Coverage Determinations: An International Comparative Study*. Maidenhead: Open University Press.

Kammen, D.M. (1995) Cookstoves for the Developing World, *Scientific American*, 273: 72–5.

Karki, D., Mirzoev, T., Green, A., Newell, J. and Baral, S. (2007) Costs of a successful public-private partnership for TB control in an urban setting in Nepal, *BMC Public Health*, 7(84): doi:10.1186/471-2458-7-84.

Kaul, I., Conceicao, P., Le Goulven, K. and Mendoza, R. (2003) *Providing Global Public Goods: Managing Globalization*. New York: Oxford University Press.

Kelley, E., Arispe, I. and Holmes, J. (2006) Beyond the initial indicators: lessons from the OECD health care quality indicators project and the US national healthcare quality report, *International Journal for Quality in Health Care*, 18: 45–51.

Kenny, N. and Chafe, R. (2007) Pushing right against evidence: turbulent times for Canadian health care, *Hastings Center Report*, 37(5): 24–6.

King, A. (2000) *The New Zealand Health Strategy*. Wellington: Ministry of Health.

King, A. (2001) *The Primary Health Care Strategy*. Wellington: Ministry of Health.

Klass, D. (2007) A performance-based conception of competence is changing the regulation of physicians' professional behavior, *Academic Medicine*, 82(6): 529–35.

Klein, R. (2007) The New Model NHS: performance, perceptions and expectations, *British Medical Bulletin*, 81–2(1): 39–50.

Kmietowicz, Z. (2003) Star rating system fails to reduce variation, *British Medical Journal*, 327: 184.

Knottnerus, J.A. and ten Velden, G.H.M. (2007) Dutch doctors and their patients: effects of health care reform in the Netherlands, *New England Journal of Medicine*, 357(24): 2424–6.

Kuperman, G.J., Spurr, C., Flammini, S. et al. (2000) A clinical information systems strategy for a large integrated delivery network, *Journal of the American Medical Informatics Association*, 7(5): 438–42.

Kwon, S. (2005) South Korea, in R. Gauld (ed.) *Comparative Health Policy in the Asia-Pacific*. Maidenhead: Open University Press.

Lalonde, M. (1974) *A New Perspective on the Health of Canadians*. Ottawa, Ontario: Ministry of Supply and Services.

Lamb, R.M., Studdert, D.M., Bohmer, R.M.J., Berwick, D. and Brennan, T.A. (2003) Hospital disclosure practices: results of a national survey, *Health Affairs*, 22(2): 73–83.

Lawson, K.A., Gregory, A.T. and Van Der Weyden, M.B. (2005) The medical colleges of Australia: beseiged but bearing up, *Medical Journal of Australia*, 183 (11/12): 646–51.

Lean, M., Lara, J. and Hill, J.O. (2006) Strategies for preventing obesity, *British Medical Bulletin*, 333: 959–62.

Leape, L., Lawthers, A.G., Brennan, T.A. and Johnson, W.G. (1993) Preventing medical injury, *Quality Review Bulletin*, 19(5): 144–9.

Lee, S.Y., Chun, C.B., Lee, Y.G. and Seo, N.K. (2008) The National Health insurance system as one type of new typology: the case of South Korea and Taiwan, *Health Policy*, 85(1): 105–13.

Leeder, S., Raymond, S., Greenberg, H., Liu, H. and Esson, K. (2004) *A Race Against Time: The Challenge of Cardiovascular Disease in Developing Economies*. New York: Earth Institute, Columbia University.

Lega, F. and Vendramini, E. (2008) Budgeting and performance management in the Italian national health system: assessment and constructive criticism, *Journal of Health Organization and Management*, 22(1): 11–22.

Leijonhufvud, A. (1968) *On Keynesian Economics and the Economics of Keynes: A Study in Monetary Theory*. Oxford: Oxford University Press.

Leonard, M., Graham, S. and Bonacum, D. (2004) The human factor: the critical importance of effective teamwork and communication in providing safe care, *Quality and Safety in Health Care*, 13(Suppl 1): i85–i90.

Liang, B.A. (2002) A system of medical error disclosure, *Quality and Safety in Health Care*, 11: 64–8.

Lisac, M. (2006) Health care reform in Germany: not the Big Bang, *Health Policy Monitor*, Survey no 8 (November).

Litva, A., Coast, J., Donovan, J., et al. (2002) 'The public is too subjective': public involvement at different levels of health-care decision making, *Social Science & Medicine*, 54: 1825–37.

Local Government Association Health Commission (2008) *Who's Accountable for Health? LGA Health Commission Final Report*. London: Local Government Association.

Long, S.K. (2008) On the road to universal coverage: impacts of reform in Massachusetts at one year, *Health Affairs*, 27: w270–w84.

McDonagh, M. (2002) E-government in Australia: the challenge of privacy of personal information, *International Journal of Law and Information Technology*, 10(3): 327–37.

McGlynn, E.A., Asch, S.M., Adams, J., et al. (2003) The quality of care delivered to adults in the United States, *New England Journal of Medicine*, 348: 2635–45.

Macintyre, S. (1997) The Black Report and beyond: what are the issues? *Social Science & Medicine*, 44(6): 723–45.

McKee, M, and Healy, J, (eds) (2002) *Hospitals in a Changing Europe*. Buckingham: Open University Press.

Mackenbach, J.P. and Bakker, M.J. (2003) Tackling socioeconomic inequalities in health: analysis of European experiences, *The Lancet*, 362: 1409–14.

McKeown, T. (1979) *The Role of Medicine: Dream, Mirage or Nemesis*. Oxford: Basil Blackwell.

McLaughlin, C. and Kaluzny, A.D. (2005) *Continuous Quality Improvement in Health Care*. Boston: Jones and Bartlett.

McMichael, A.J., Powles, J.W., Butler, C.D. and Uauy, R. (2007) Food, livestock production, energy, climate change, and health, *The Lancet*, 370: 1253–63.

McNeill, P., Kerridge, I., Arcuili, C., et al. (2006) Gifts, drug samples, and other items given to medical specialists by pharmaceutical companies, *Journal of Bioethical Inquiry*, 3(3): 139–48.

Malcolm, L. and Mays, N. (1999) New Zealand's independent practitioner associations: a working model of clinical governance in primary care? *British Medical Journal*, 319: 1340–2.

Malcolm, L., Wright, L., Barnett, P. and Hendry, C. (2002) *Clinical Leadership and Quality in Primary Care Organisations in New Zealand: Report commissioned by the Clinical Leaders Association of New Zealand for the Ministry of Health*. Auckland: Clinical Leaders Association of New Zealand.

Malcolm, L., Wright, L., Barnett, P. and Hendry, C. (2003) Building a successful partnership between management and clinical leadership: experience from New Zealand, *British Medical Journal*, 326: 653–4.

Mannion, R., Davies, H. and Marshall, M. (2005) Impact of star performance ratings in English acute hospital trusts, *Journal of Health Services Research and Policy*, 10(1): 18–24.

Marmot, M., and Richardson, R. (eds) (2005) *Social Determinants of Health, 2nd Edn*. New York: Oxford University Press.

Marmot, M., Smith, G.D., Stansfeld, S., et al. (1991) Health inequalities among British civil servants: the Whitehall II study, *The Lancet*, 337: 1387–93.

Martin, J. and Begg, E. (2000) Reference pricing: is it in the public interest? *New Zealand Medical Journal*, 113: 422–4.

Mays, N. (2008) Origins and development of the National Health Service, in G. Scambler (ed.) *Sociology as Applied to Medicine, Sixth Edn*. London: Elsevier.

Meehan, T.P., Wang, Y., Tate, J.P., et al. (2006) Improving the quality of preventive cardiovascular care provided by primary care physicians: insights from a US quality improvement organization, *International Journal for Quality in Health Care*, 18(3): 186–94.

Mehrotra, A., Epstein, A.M. and Rosenthal, M.B. (2006) Do integrated medical groups provide higher-quality medical care than individual practice associations?, *Annals of Internal Medicine*, 145: 826–33.

Mello, M. and Joffe, S. (2007) Compact versus contract: industry sponsors' obligations to their research subjects, *New England Journal of Medicine*, 356 (26): 2737–43.

Merry, A. and Seddon, M. (2006) Quality improvement in healthcare in New Zealand. Part 2: Are our patients safe – and what are we doing about it?, *New Zealand Medical Journal*, 119(1238): 1–7.

Miller, R.H. and Sim, I. (2004) Physicians' use of electronic medical records: barriers and solutions, *Health Affairs*, 23(2): 116–26.

Milner, H. (1990) *Sweden: Social Democracy in Practice*. Oxford: Oxford University Press.

Ministry of Health (2007) *Health Targets: Moving Towards Healthier Futures 2007/08*. Wellington: Ministry of Health.

Ministry of Health (2008) *DHB Hospital Benchmark Information*.

Report for the Quarter April–June 2008. Wellington: Ministry of Health.

Ministry of Health (2006) *Implementing the New Zealand Health Strategy 2006*. Wellington: Ministry of Health.

Mitchell, W. and Simmons, R. (1994) *Beyond Politics: Markets, Welfare, and the Failure of Bureaucracy*. Boulder, CA: Westview Press.

Moran, M. (1994) Reshaping the health-care state, *Government and Opposition*, 29(1): 48–63.

Mossialos, E. and Dixon, A. (2002) Funding health care: an introduction, in E. Mossialos, A. Dixon, J. Figueras and J. Kutzin (eds) *Funding Health Care: Options for Europe*. Buckingham: Open University Press.

Mossialos, E., Dixon, A., Figueras, J. and Kutzin, J. (eds) (2002) *Funding Health Care: Options for Europe*. Buckingham: Open University Press.

Moynihan, R. (2008) The invisible influence, *British Medical Journal*, 336: 417.

Munn, J. and Wozniak, L. (2007) Single-payer health care systems: the roles and responsibilities of the public and private sectors, *Benefits Quarterly*, 23 (3): 7–16.

Murray, E., Lo, B., Pollack, L., et al. (2003) The impact of health information on the Internet on the physician-patient relationship: patient perceptions, *Archives of Internal Medicine*, 163: 1727–34.

Nancarrow, S.A. and Borthwick, A.M. (2005) Dynamic professional boundaries in the healthcare workforce, *Sociology of Health and Illness*, 27: 897–919.

Nathan, S.A., Develin, E., Grove, N. and Zwi, A. (2005) An Australian childhood obesity summit: the role of data and evidence in 'public' policy making, *Australia and New Zealand Health Policy*, 2(17):dio: 10.1186/743–8462–2–17.

National Association of Community Health Centers (2008) *Access Transformed: Building a Primary Care Workforce for the 21st Century*. Bethesda MD: National Association of Community Health Centers.

National Audit Office. 2006. *Department of Health. The National Programme for IT in the NHS*. London: National Audit Office.

National Health Committee (1998) *The Social, Economic and Cultural Determinants of Health in New Zealand*. Wellington: National Health Committee.

National Health Information Management Advisory Council (1999) *Health Online: A Health Information Action Plan for Australia*.

Canberra: National Health Information Management Advisory Council.

Navarro, V. (ed.) (2007) *Neoliberalism, Globalization and Inequalities: Consequences for Health and Quality of Life.* Amityville, NY: Baywood Publishing Company.

Navarro, V. and Shi, L. (2001) The political context of social inequalities and health, *International Journal of Health Services*, 31(1): 1–21.

NHS Connecting for Health (2007) *Costs for NHS National Programme for Information Technology Implementation.* London: NHS Connecting for Health www.connectingforhealth.nhs.uk/newsroom/news-stories/131004.

NHS Executive (1998) *Information for Health: An Information Strategy for the Modern NHS 1998–2005.* West Yorkshire: Department of Health Publications.

Nicholls, S., Cullen, R., O'Neill, S. and Halligan, A. (2000) Clinical governance: its origins and its foundations, *British Journal of Clinical Governance*, 5(3): 172–8.

Nichols, L.M., Ginsberg, P.B., Berenson, R.A., et al. (2004) Are market forces strong enough to deliver efficient health care systems? Confidence is waning, *Health Affairs*, 23(2): 8–21.

Norris, A.C. (2002) *Essentials of Telemedicine and Telecare.* Chichester: Wiley and Co.

Oberlander, J. (2002) The US health care system: on a road to nowhere?, *Canadian Medical Association Journal*, 167(2): 163–8.

Oberlander, J. (2003) *The Political Life of Medicare.* Chicago: University of Chicago Press.

O'Brien, M. (2008) *Poverty, Policy and the State: The Changing Face of Social Security.* Bristol: The Policy Press.

O'Connor, A.M., Stacey, D. and Legare, F. (2008) Coaching to support patients in making decisions, *British Medical Journal*, 336: 228–9.

OECD (2007) *Health at a Glance 2007.* Paris: OECD.

OECD (2008a) *OECD Health Data.* Paris: OECD.

OECD (2008b) *The Looming Crisis of the Health Workforce: How Can OECD Countries Respond?* Paris: OECD.

Oliver, A. (2007) Inconsistent objectives: reflections on some selective health care policy developments in Europe, *Health Economics, Policy and Law*, 2: 93–106.

Oliver, A. (2008) Public-sector health-care reforms that work? A case study of the US veterans health administration, *The Lancet*, 371: 1211–13.

Olson, M. (1965) *The Logic of Collective Action: Public Goods and the Theory of Groups*. Cambridge, MA: Harvard University Press.

Pagliari, C., Detmer, D. and Singleton, P. (2007) Potential of electronic personal health records, *British Medical Journal*, 335: 330–3.

Paterson, R. (2002) The patients' complaints system in New Zealand, *Health Affairs*, 21(3): 70–9.

Paterson, W.E.T. and Thomas, A.H. (eds) (1986) *The Future of Social Democracy: Problems and Prospects of Social Democratic Parties in Western Europe*. Oxford: Oxford University Press.

Paul, C., Nicholls, R., Priest, P. and McGee, R. (2008) Making policy decisions about population screening for breast cancer: the role of citizens' deliberation, *Health Policy*, 85: 314–20.

Peters, B.G. and Pierre, J. (1998) Governance without government? Rethinking public administration, *Journal of Public Administration Research and Theory*, 8(2): 223–43.

Peterson, A. and Lupton, D. (1996) *The New Public Health: Health and Self in the Age of Risk*. St Leonards, NSW: Allen and Unwin.

Pickett, K.E. and Wilkinson, R.G. (2007) Child well-being and income inequality in rich societies: ecological cross sectional study, *British Medical Journal*, 335(1080): doi:10.1136/bmj.39377.580162.55.

Pollock, A.M. and Godden, S. (2008) Independent sector treatment centres: evidence so far, *British Medical Journal*, 336: 421–4.

Quam, L., Smith, R. and Yach, D. (2006) Rising to the global challenge of the chronic disease epidemic, *The Lancet*, 368: 1221–3.

Quaye, R.K. (2007) Is the Swedish welfare state in retreat? Current trends in Swedish health care, *International Journal of Health Care Quality Assurance*, 20(5): 392–404.

Raine, R., Sanderson, C. and Black, N. (2005) Developing clinical guidelines: a challenge to current methods, *British Medical Journal*, 331: 631–3.

Ranade, W. (ed.) (1998) *Markets and Health Care: A Comparative Analysis*. London: Longman.

Rawlins, M. (1999) In pursuit of quality: the National Institute for Clinical Excellence, *The Lancet*, 353(9158): 1079–82.

Reeves, G.K., Pirie, K.P., Beral, V., et al. (2007) Cancer incidence and mortality in relation to body mass index in the million women study: cohort study, *British Medical Journal*, 335: 1134–45.

Reiser, S.J. and Banner, R.S. (2003) The charter on medical professionalism and the limits of medical power, *Annals of Internal Medicine*, 138(10): 844–6.

Rhodes, R.A.W. (1997) *Understanding Governance: Policy Networks, Governance, Reflexivity and Accountability*. Buckingham: Open University Press.

Rifkin, S.B. (1981) The role of the public in the planning, management and evaluation of health activities and programmes, including self-care, *Social Science & Medicine*, 15A: 377–86.

Rifkin, S.B. and Walt, G. (1986) Why health improves: defining the issues concerning 'Comprehensive Primary Health Care' and 'Selective Primary Health Care', *Social Science & Medicine*, 6: 559–66.

Rittenhouse, D.R., Casilino, L., Gilles, R., Shortell, S.M. and Lau, B. (2008) Measuring the medical home infrastructure in large medical groups, *Health Affairs*, 27(5): 1246–58.

Rose, R. (1993) *Lesson Drawing in Public Policy*. New Jersey: Chatham House.

Rosenthal, M.B., Fernandopulle, R., HyunSook, R.S. and Landon, B. (2004) Paying for quality: providers' incentives for quality improvement, *Health Affairs*, 23(2): 127–41.

Rosenthal, M.B., Landon, B., Normand, S.T., Frank, R.G. and Epstein, A.M. (2006) Pay for performance in commercial HMOs, *New England Journal of Medicine*, 355: 1895–902.

Royal Academy of Engineering and British Computer Society (2004) *The Challenges of Complex IT Projects*. London: The Royal Academy of Engineering.

Salisbury, C. (2008) The involvement of private companies in NHS general practice, *British Medical Journal*, 336: 400–1.

Salter, B. (2007) Governing UK medical performance: the struggle for policy dominance, *Health Policy*, 82: 263–75.

Saltman, R.B., Busse, R. and Figueras, J. (eds) (2004) *Social Health Insurance Systems in Western Europe*. Maidenhead: Open University Press.

Saltman, R.B. and Ferroussier-Davis, O. (2000) The concept of stewardship in health policy, *Bulletin of the World Health Organization*, 78(6): 732–9.

Saltman, R.B., Rico, A. and Boerma, W. (eds) (2006) *Primary Care in the Driver's Seat? Organizational Reform in European Primary Care*. Maidenhead: Open University Press.

Scally, G. and Donaldson, L. (1998) Clinical governance and the drive for quality improvement in the new NHS in England, *British Medical Journal*, 317(7150): 61–5.

Schade, C.P., Sullivan, F.M., Lusignan, S. and Madeley, J. (2006) e-prescribing, efficiency, quality: lessons from the computerization of UK family practice, *Journal of the American Medical Informatics Association*, 13(5): 470–5.

Schneider, E.C., Zaslavsky, A.M. and Epstein, A.M. (2005) Quality of care in for-profit and not-for-profit health plans enrolling Medicare beneficiaries, *American Journal of Medicine*, 118(12): 1392–400.

Scott, C. (2001) *Public and Private Roles in Health Care Systems: Reform Experiences in Seven OECD Countries*. Buckingham: Open University Press.

Secretary of State for the Environment, Food and Rural Affairs (2006) *Climate Change: The UK Programme 2006*. London: HMSO.

Selin, H. and VanDeveer, S.D. (2007) Political science and prediction: what's next for US climate change policy? *Review of Policy Research*, 24(1): 1–27.

Shapiro, J. and Smith, S. (2003) Lessons for the NHS from Kaiser Permanente, *British Medical Journal*, 237: 1241–2.

Shaw, K., MacKillop, L. and Armitage, M. (2007) Revalidation, appraisal and clinical governance, *Clinical Governance: An International Journal*, 12(3): 170–7.

Shipman Inquiry (2004) *Fifth Report – Safeguarding Patients: Lessons from the Past – Proposals for the Future*. London: The Shipman Inquiry.

Shiwani, M.H. (2006) Clinical governance in Pakistan: myth or reality?' *Journal of the Pakistan Medical Association*, 56(3): 94–5.

Shoen, C., Osborn, R., Huynh, P.T., et al. (2006) On the front lines of care: primary care doctors' office systems, experiences, and views in seven countries, *Health Affairs*, 25: w555–w71.

Siciliani, L. and Hurst, J. (2005) Tackling excessive waiting times for elective surgery: a comparative analysis of policies in 12 OECD countries, *Health Policy*, 72(2): 201–15.

Signal, L., Martin, J., Reid, P., et al. (2007) Tackling health inequalities: moving theory to action, *International Journal for Equity in Health*, 6(12): doi:10.1186/475–9276–6–12.

Smedley, B.D. (2008) Moving beyond access: achieving equity in state health reform, *Health Affairs*, 27(2): 447–55.

Smith, J. (2000) *Health Management Information Systems: A Handbook for Decisionmakers*. Buckingham: Open University Press.

Smith, P.C. and Goddard, M. (2000) Reforming health care markets, in P. C. Smith (ed.) *Reforming Markets in Health Care*. Buckingham: Open University Press.

Socha, K. and Bech, M. (2007) Extended free choice of hospital – waiting time, *Health Policy Monitor*, Survey 10 (October).

Som, C.V. (2007) Exploring the human resource implications of clinical governance, *Health Policy*, 80: 281–96.

Standish Group (2001) *Extreme Chaos*. Boston: The Standish Group International, Inc.

Starfield, B., Shi, L. and Macinko, J. (2005) Contribution of primary care to health systems and health, *The Milbank Quarterly*, 83(3): 457–502.

Stent, R. (1998) *Canterbury Health Limited: A Report by the Health and Disability Commissioner April*. Wellington: Health and Disability Commissioner.

Strandberg-Larsen, M., Neilsen, M.B., Vallgarda, S., Krasnik, A. and Vrangbaek, K. (2007) *Denmark: Health System Review*. Copenhagen: European Union Observatory on Health Systems and Policies.

Suhrcke, M., McKee, M. and Rocco, L. (2007) Health investment benefits economic development, *The Lancet*, 370: 1467–8.

Sussex, J. (2003) Public-private partnerships in hospital development: lessons from the UK's 'Private Finance Initiative', *Research in Healthcare Financial Management*, 8(1): 59–76.

Swinburne, B., Caterson, I., Seidell, J.C. and James, W.P.T. (2004) Diet, nutrition and the prevention of excess weight gain and obesity, *Public Health Nutrition*, 7(1a): 123–46.

Swinburne, B., Milne, R., Richards, M., et al. (2000) Reimbursement of pharmaceuticals in New Zealand: comments on Pharmac's processes, *New Zealand Medical Journal*, 113: 425–7.

Szreter, S. (1988) The importance of social intervention in Britain's mortality decline ca.1850–1914: a reinterpretation of the role of public health, *The Society for the Social History of Medicine*, 1(1): 1–37.

Tang, H. and Ng, J.H.K. (2006) Googling for a diagnosis – use of Google as a diagnostic aid: Internet based study, *British Medical Journal*, 333: 1143–5.

Tang, P.C., Ash, J.S., Bates, D.W., Overhage, J.M. and Sands, D.Z. (2006) Personal health records: definitions, benefits, and strategies for overcoming barriers to adoption, *Journal of the American Medical Informatics Association*, 13(2): 121–6.

Tanser, F.C., Sharp, B. and le Sueur, D. (2003) Potential effect of climate change on malaria transmission in Africa, *The Lancet*, 362: 1792–8.

Taylor, I. (2000) New Labour and the enabling State, *Health and Social Care in the Community*, 8(6): 372–9.

Tesh, S.N. (1995) Miasma and 'social factors' in disease causality: lessons from the ninteenth century, *Journal of Health Politics, Policy and Law*, 20(4): 1001–24.

Thomas, E.J., Studdert, D.M., Burstin, H.R., et al. (2000) Incidence and types of adverse events and negligent care in Utah and Colorado, *Medical Care*, 38(3): 247–9.

Thompson, A.G.H. (2007) The meaning of patient involvement and participation in health care consultations: a taxonomy, *Social Science & Medicine*, 64: 1297–310.

Thompson, G., Frances, J., Levacic, R. and Mitchell, J. (eds) (1991) *Markets, Hierarchies and Networks: The Coordination of Social Life*. London: Sage.

Thomson, S. and Dixon, A. (2006) Choices in health care: the European experience, *Journal of Health Services Research and Policy*, 11(3): 167–71.

Timmins, N. (2005a) Challenges of private provision in the NHS, *British Medical Journal*, 331: 1193–5.

Timmins, N. (2005b) Use of private health care in the NHS, *British Medical* Journal, 331: 1141–2.

Trouiller, P., Olliaro, P., Torreele, E., et al. (2002) Drug development for neglected diseases: a deficient market and a public-health policy failure, *The Lancet*, 359: 2188–94.

Tuohy, C.H., Flood, C.M. and Stabile, M. (2004) How does private finance affect public health care systems? Marshaling the evidence from OECD nations, *Journal of Health Politics, Policy and Law*, 29(3): 359–96.

UNAIDS (2006) *2006 Report on the Global AIDS Epidemic*. Geneva: UNAIDS.

United Nations Development Programme (2007) *The Millennium Development Goals Report 2007*. New York: United Nations.

United States Congress (2005) Patient safety and quality Improvement Act of 2005, 109th Congress.

US Department of Health and Human Services (1998) *Healthy People 2010: Understanding and Improving Health*. Washington DC: Department of Health and Human Services.

Valimaki, M., Nenonen, H., Koivunen, M. and Suhonen, R. (2007) Patients' perceptions of Internet usage and their opportunity to obtain health information, *Medical Informatics and the Internet in Medicine*, 32(3): 305–14.

van Ginneken, E. (2006) Health insurance reform in the Netherlands, *Health Policy Monitor*, Survey no 6 (March).

Vincent, C., Neale, G. and Woloshynowych, M. (2001) Adverse

events in British hospitals: preliminary retrospective record review, *British Medical Bulletin*, 322: 517–19.

Vrangbaek, K. (2008) Public–private partnerships in the health sector: the Danish experience, *Health Economics, Policy and Law*, 3: 141–63.

Wait, S. and Nolte, E. (2006) Public involvement policies in health: exploring their conceptual basis, *Health Economics, Policy and Law*, 1: 149–62.

Walsh, K. (1995) *Public Services and Market Mechanisms: Competition, Contracting and the New Public Management*. London: Macmillan.

Walt, G. and Buse, K. (2006) Global cooperation in international public health, in M. Merson, R.E. Black and A. Mills (eds) *International Public Health: Diseases, Programs, Systems, and Policies*. Boston: Jones and Bartlett.

Waring, J. (2007) Adaptive regulation or governmentality: patient safety and the changing regulation of medicine, *Sociology of Health and Illness*, 29(2): 163–79.

WAVE Advisory Board (2001) *From Strategy to Reality: The WAVE Project*. Wellington: Ministry of Health.

Weingart, S.N., Pagovich, O., Sands, D.Z., et al. (2005) What can hospitalized patients tell us about adverse events? Learning from patient-reported incidents, *Journal of General Internal Medicine*, 20(9): 830–6.

Wennberg, J.E. (1999) Understanding geographical variations in health care delivery, *New England Journal of Medicine*, 340: 52–3.

Wermuth, L. (2003) *Global Inequality and Human Needs: Health and Illness in an Increasingly Unequal World*. Boston: Pearson Education.

Widdus, R. (2005) Public–private partnerships: an overview, *Journal of the Royal Society of Tropical Medicine and Hygiene*, 99s: s1–s8.

Wilkinson, R. (2005) *The Impact of Inequality: How to Make Sick Societies Healthier*. New York: The New Press.

Wilkinson, R., and Marmot, M. (2003) *Social Determinant of Health: The Solid Facts, 2nd edn*. Copenhagen: World Health Organization, Regional Office for Europe.

Williams, S.K. and Osborn, S.S. (2006) The development of the national reporting and learning system in England and Wales, 2001–2006, *Medical Journal of Australia* 184(10): s65–s8.

Wilsford, D. (1994) Path dependency, or why history makes it difficult but not impossible to reform health systems in a big way, *Journal of Public Policy*, 4(13): 251–83.

Wilson, J.Q. (1989) *Bureaucracy: What Government Agencies Do and Why They Do It*. New York: Basic Books.

Wilson, R.M., Runciman, W.B., Gibberd, R.W., et al. (1995) The quality in Australian health care study, *Medical Journal of Australia*, 163: 458–71.

Woodward, A. and Kawachi, I. (2000) Why reduce health inequalities?, *Journal of Epidemiology and Community Health* 54: 923–9.

Woolf, S., Grol, R., Hutchinson, A., Eccles, M. and Grimshaw, J. (1999) Potential benefits, limitations, and harms of clinical guidelines, *British Medical Journal*, 318: 527–30.

Woolhandler, S. and Himmelstein, D. (2007) Competition in a publicly funded healthcare system, *British Medical Journal*, 335: 1126–9.

World Health Organization (1978) *Alma-Ata Declaration on Primary Healthcare: Report of the International Conference on Primary Health Care*. Geneva: World Health Organization.

World Health Organization (1986) Ottawa Charter for Health Promotion, *Health Promotion*, 1(4): i–v.

World Health Organization (2005) *Preventing Chronic Diseases: A Vital Investment*. Geneva: World Health Organization.

World Health Organization (1997) *The Jakarta Declaration on Leading Health Promotion into the 21st Century*. Geneva: World Health Organization.

World Health Organization (2006) *The World Health Report 2006: Working Together for Health*. Geneva: World Health Organization.

World Health Organization (2007) *World Health Statistics 2006*. Geneva: World Health Organization.

World Health Organization (2008) *The World Health Report 2008: Primary Health Care – Now More Than Ever*. Geneva: World Health Organization.

World Resources Institute (2006) *Climate and Atmosphere: Country Profile – United States*. Washington, DC: World Bank.

Wright, A.A. and Katz, I.T. (2005) Bar coding for patient safety, *New England Journal of Medicine*, 353(4): 329–31.

Wu, A.W.W. (1999) Handling hospital errors: is disclosure the best defense?, *Annals of Internal Medicine*. 131(12): 970–2.

Yach, D., Hawkes, C., Epping-Jordan, J.E. and Steyn, K. (2006) Chronic diseases and risks, in M. Merson, R.E. Black and A. Mills (eds) *International Public Health: Diseases, Programs, Systems and Policies*. Sudbury, MA: Jones and Bartlett.

Yoon, K.H., Lee, J.H., Kim, J.W., et al. (2006) Epidemic obesity and type 2 diabetes in Asia, *The Lancet*, 368: 1681–8.

Zhou, Y.Y., Garrido, T., Chin, H.L., Wiesenthal, A.M. and Liang, L.L. (2007) Patient access to an electronic health record with secure messaging: impact on primary care utilization, *American Journal of Managed Care*, 13: 418–24.

Author Index

Subject Index

A number in **bold** indicates a figure, table, or boxed topic. An en dash (–) between two numbers indicates continuous treatment of a topic, a tilde (~) only that a topic is referred to on each page in the range.

Related books from Open University Press

Puchase from www.openup.co.uk or order through your local bookseller

---

TRUST MATTERS IN HEALTH CARE

Michael Calnan and Rosemary Rowe

- Does trust still matter in health care and who does it matter to?
- Have trust relations changed in the 'New' NHS?
- What does trust mean to patients, clinicians and managers?

In the NHS trust has traditionally played an important part in the relationships between its three key actors: the state, health care practitioners and patients. However, in recent years the environments in which these relationships operate have been subject to considerable change as the NHS has been modernised. Patients are now expected to play a more active role, both in self-managing their illness and in choice of care provider and clinicians are expected to work in teams and in partnership with managers. This unique book explores the importance of trust, how it is lost and won and the extent to which trust relationships in health care may have changed. The book combines theoretical and empirical analysis, while also examining the role of policy.

Calnan and Rowe analyse data collected from interviews with patients, health care professionals and managers in primary care and acute care settings. Among the issues covered are:

- The importance of trust to their relationships
- What constitutes high and low trust behaviour
- The changing nature of trust relations between patients, clinicians and managers
- How trust can be built and sustained
- How interpersonal trust affects institutional trust

Trust Matters in Health Care is key reading for policy makers, health care professionals and managers in the public and private sector, and a useful resource for educators and students within health and social care and management studies.

Contents

Series editor's introduction - Preface - Acknowledgements - Trust in the context of healthcare - Trust in the NHS: Theoretical perspectives - Trust between patients and clinicians - Trust between clinicians - Trust relations between clinicians, managers and patients - Trust still matters in healthcare? - Appendix: Case study selection and methods - Case study 1: Diabetes - Case study 2: Hip surgery - References - Index.

2008 224pp
978–0–335–22283–4 (Paperback)   978–0–335–22284–1 (Hardback)

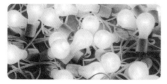 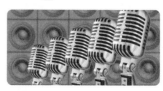
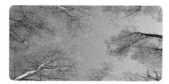 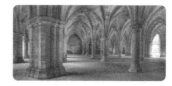
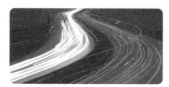 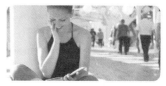
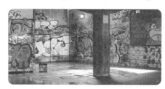